Calm Seas

Keys to the Successful Treatment of Bipolar Disorder

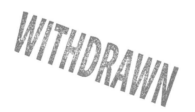

Calm Seas

Keys to the Successful Treatment of Bipolar Disorder

Roger Sparhawk, M.D.

CreateSpace
an Amazon Company

Table of Contents

Dedication

This book is dedicated to the patients and their families and loved ones,

to the next generation of clinicians who will be treating patients
with mood disorders,

and to the late J. Patrick Duffy, M.D.,

Residency Training Director at University Hospitals of Cleveland,
who trained as a psychoanalyst and then as a mood specialist,
and who then worked diligently with patients and their loved ones
at the interface
of psychotherapy and the mood disorders.

Introduction:

The Goal:

We have the opportunity to help 5 million people,
patients with bipolar disorder
and their families and loved ones,
to achieve a substantially higher quality of life.

There are about 309 million people in the United States alone,[217] of whom approximately 3% to 4% suffer with bipolar disorder.[1,45,55,183] That's about 10 million people with bipolar disorder. Perhaps half of them are getting some form of treatment, which would be almost 5 million individuals. At least half of these have failed to reach stable recovery, that is, about 2 ½ million people. The illness and its effects in each bipolar patient have seriously damaged the life quality of at least 1 other person, and usually far more than that, and so, between the patients and those close to them, the number of people who stand to benefit substantially from an improvement in the real-world applied treatment of bipolar disorder is at least 5 million people. It is this group whose quality of life we aim to improve.

Just stop and take this idea in and think about it a moment: We can substantially improve the quality of life of 5 million people. Should we seize this opportunity?

This book is a guide to help us reach this goal. In it I attempt to explain the available scientific literature on bipolar disorder treatment in a way that most people can understand.

Especially if this condition affects you or your loved ones, please read on.

How to Read this Book

In the book, I try to include enough references (marked by the small raised numbers, like[1]) so that if you want to, you can look things up and decide for yourself. You will also find some small raised letters, which refer to explanations in footnotes at the bottom of the page. Further explanations of some of the terms and abbreviations may be found in the Glossary at the back of the book. The Appendix is right after the Glossary and contains diagnostic criteria of numerous disorders according to the official diagnostic manual of the American Psychiatric Association, the DSM-IV-TR.[24] The diagnostic criteria include the sets of symptoms required to make a diagnosis of a specific psychiatric disorder according to the manual. You can also look up additional information on our website, www.calmseas.us.

Disclaimer

This book is meant to serve as a teaching device only. I have reviewed the information in the following chapters to try to make sure that it is accurate, but accuracy can't be guaranteed. There are also honest differences of opinion, so what seems correct to me might well be seen somewhat differently by someone else.

The information in this book applies primarily to those with an accurate and reliably-determined diagnosis of bipolar I or bipolar II disorder, as the findings of the clinical research on other bipolar conditions are far less clear.[184,185]

If you wonder whether or not you have bipolar disorder, I would also recommend the excellent book by Jim Phelps, M.D., *Why Am I Still Depressed?*

It is my opinion that patients and their support people who become more actively involved in their treatment tend to do better. Please remember, however, that your own treatment needs to be planned with and managed by your own healthcare provider.

Acknowledgements

I want to acknowledge and thank:

Roy Chengappa, M.D., for his encouragement for this project.

S. Nassir Ghaemi, M.D., M.P.H., his consistent writing, teaching, mentoring and collaboration over the years, and especially for providing a workable model for the treatment of bipolar disorder, which, starting in 2001, helped the whole thing start to make sense again.

Neisha DeSouza, M.D., and Clara Ruiz, M.D., and the psychiatric residents with whom I've worked over the years, for their inspiration via the curiosity and enormous potential of psychiatrists in training.

Charles L. Bowden, M.D., for his observations about psychiatric residency training, for his helpful review of early chapters, and for his encouragement for the need for additional understandable information and explanations for patients and their families.

Bijan Bastani, M.D., for providing many insights into the process of clinical trials design and the workings of clinical trials, for mentoring me as a clinical trials investigator, and for acquainting me with the MINI-D, a remarkable screening diagnostic instrument with implications for what's possible.

My gifted and accomplished supervisors at University Hospitals of Cleveland, the Cleveland Psychoanalytic Institute, and the Cleveland Veterans Administration Hospital, who repeatedly reminded me to "Listen to your patients; they'll tell you everything you need to know."

The University of Chicago Psychiatric Board Review Course, for teaching me how one can arrive at a credible diagnostic formulation in the first interview.

Stephen M. Stahl, M.D., Ph.D., for providing an understandable view of the mechanisms of action of numerous psychotropic medications, for modeling the successful presentation methods of the well-trained psychiatric speaker and teacher, and for providing me the remarkable opportunity to train with and work for the Neuroscience Education Institute (NEI) providing regional continuing medical education programs.

Rick Davis, Ph.D., and his talented cadre of professional speaker trainers, for providing exceptional speaker training in collaboration with NEI, and for providing critical insights into the many important facets of adult learning.

Susan A. Duppstadt, M.D., for serving as the highly capable Editor in Chief.

Elissa Folk, for her skilled and artistic graphics renderings, including the beautiful covers.

Todd Ivan, M.D., for his helpful review of early chapters, and steady encouragement for the project.

Deanna Horrigan, R.N., CNS, for her tenacious review of almost all chapters of the book, and her courage in testing these now nearly forgotten but highly effective ideas in practice.

Kim Sweeney, for serving as librarian extraordinaire for clinical research questions during much of the process.

Karen McCroskey, for her very gracious support and appreciation, and for her steadfast enthusiasm for this project.

Phebe Simpson, R.N., for her help in reviewing book chapters and consistently encouraging the work of this project.

Monica Halter, R.N., C.N.P., for her interest, encouragement, and for helping us find our very capable graphic designer.

Chris France, Psy.D., for his insights into, and collaboration on clinical research.

Joan Wilson, Ph.D., for her considerable interest in bipolar disorder, and for her skill in collaborating with me in the care of numerous patients with the disorder.

Susan Jones and her nurse practitioner students at Kent State University, for their collaboration on clinical research.

Those contributors I may have forgotten to mention; my apologies.

And to those many others, including patients, families, and clinicians, who provided so much in the way of personal experience with bipolar disorder and eagerness to help provide better outcomes for others going forward.

Section A:

Understanding the Broad Issues

Chapter 1

Why I'm Writing This Book

Bipolar disorder (BD) holds the dubious distinction of being one of the most complex conditions faced in psychiatric practice.[2]

Simplicity is the key to complexity.[3]

As the first quote and many other descriptions point out, bipolar disorder is in some ways very complex. Seen from a different viewpoint, however, it is extremely simple.

As we get started, I'll discuss with you three examples of some of the parts of the puzzle that make bipolar disorder much easier to understand.

First, viewing it as a puzzle rather than as a monster helps us relax, focus better, and even have some fun sorting all this out. I genuinely have fun sorting these puzzles out with my own bipolar patients, so I hope and believe this will make the whole process easier and more fun for you. This book aims to break the puzzle down into a number of very understandable pieces.

Second, the way bipolar disorder behaves over time seems at first glance to be very complicated. After we break it down into its parts (in Chapters 4 and 5), however, it is much simpler, and much more easily understood.

Third, on the treatment side, bipolar disorder seems to many people to be untreatable. I think you'll see in the following pages, however, that this just isn't quite so. It turns out that the treatment is actually much simpler than we may now think. Once we compare the two most common treatment approaches side by side in Chapter 3, the choices between them may prove much easier than you might have imagined.

Doctors and nurse practitioners treating bipolar disorder in the United States have received extensive training and are highly skilled. They are also dedicated to helping their patients, including their patients with bipolar disorder. Over the past several years, however, the treatment of bipolar disorder in the United States has resulted in only fair to poor outcomes when compared to the goal of stable long-term recovery with improved functioning.

This difference between known treatability and actual outcome would seem somewhat confusing, and a serious concern for those suffering the disorder. Much of the difference has to do with training. U.S. clinicians have received extensive training in the diagnosis and treatment of "regular" major depressive disorder, that is, depression with no personal history of manias ever.[a] U.S. clinicians have been provided considerably less training in the diagnosis and treatment of bipolar disorder.

Much of the training they do receive in the treatment of bipolar disorder may be with strategies and medications that aren't successful very often.

There are other strategies that I'll be describing to you as more successful. These strategies have largely been lost and forgotten over the past several years, both from treatment as usual in the community, and also from many residency training programs and nurse practitioner training programs. As a result, many clinicians may not have had exposure to, or positive experience with, the more successful strategies, and thus don't use them with their patients. So, in a sense, this book will be teaching you about what has largely become the lost art of effective bipolar disorder treatment.

Some of the difference between known treatability and disappointing outcomes may be related to what I believe to be unhelpful concepts in how our current diagnostic system distinguishes between bipolar depression and bipolar

---

a Mood specialists call this "unipolar depression" or "unipolar disorder," because the episodes have only one "pole," down, as opposed to "bipolar" disorder, which has 2 poles, up and down.

mixed episodes, and this is described in detail in Chapter 5.

Another reason has to do with the extremely powerful belief among many patients, families and clinicians in the U.S. that the medicines called "antidepressants" will help more than a very small minority of bipolar patients for more than 3 months. By contrast, the traditional mood stabilizers have been largely lost from view, in part because all their patents have expired, and they are therefore no longer actively marketed and promoted.

My own professional experience as a psychiatrist specializing in bipolar disorder is that bipolar disorder is extremely treatable, and we should routinely expect to get most patients to a stable recovery with substantial lessening of mood symptoms, with complete or near-complete clearing of major mood episodes, and with noticeable improvement in their ability to function. These good outcomes are easier to achieve if known effective treatment approaches are applied early in the course of the disorder.

I routinely tell my patients to expect a good outcome; and if they follow through with the treatment, that is what usually happens. If you promise not to tell this secret to anyone, I'll tell you a little rule that I've observed over the past 10 years or so: The bipolar disorder itself is almost[b] always treatable.

Since this rule reaches well beyond what any clinical research has been able to prove so far, and even beyond what I've seen anyone else write, I've been trying for the past several years to disprove this rule in my clinical practice. I've asked for and welcomed "treatment failures" and "tough cases" from my colleagues. I have also welcomed "impossible cases," patients who decided for some reason after years and sometimes decades of failed treatments to give treatment with another new doctor one very last try before they go for their final appointment with the coroner or undertaker.

Even with all this, I just haven't found more than a handful of people whose bipolar illness seems to contradict the above rule. If the patient and I, often together with a close family member (or members) or support person, stubbornly pursue whatever we may have missed, and whatever reasonable treatment

---

b My editor made me add "almost," because there are, infrequently, patients whose bipolar disorder just simply doesn't respond very well to reasonable treatments. On the hand, I continue to approach all my bipolar patients with the Cowpens Mentality described in Chapter 14.

approaches[4,5,6,7] we may not yet have tried, most of these patients get better also. In summary, as much as I've tried to find people with untreatable bipolar disorder, I just haven't been able to find very many.

Now sometimes I wish I could claim that this was because of personal genius, but that isn't the reason. These good results are essentially available to anyone who learns and applies the "cycling and recurrence" approach to the treatment of bipolar disorder.[4,5,6,7] This approach is well supported by scientific evidence and my own experience, and is described in more detail in Chapter 3.

We achieve good outcomes when my patients, their close loved ones, and I pay close attention to certain concepts, principles, and treatment approaches I have learned from bipolar disorder experts and specialists over the past 35 years.

When we deviate from these approaches, things fairly predictably get worse. I therefore explain to the patient and family that it is important for us to give the scientifically proven strategies solid trials before we move on to trying unproven strategies, or strategies that have been shown to fail in the vast majority of patients.

One of the goals of this book is to explain these proven concepts, principles, and approaches to you, and to contrast these with other more popular approaches which have been shown to be much more likely to fail. You should be aware that these less successful treatment approaches are nonetheless currently much more widely taught and used in the everyday clinical treatment of patients with bipolar disorder than the approaches I'll be explaining to you.

The process of describing some treatment approaches as proven, and others as having been shown to be likely to fail, is sure to stir up some controversy, but in my opinion there are some very clear, consistent, and meaningful findings in the clinical research on bipolar disorder which are not yet widely known, and certainly not widely applied by most clinicians with their own patients.[8,9,92,93]

The clinical research literature is referenced with the little raised numbers throughout the book, so that those who want to learn more can look the articles up in the reference list at the end of the book. This will allow you to read these articles and reach your own conclusions.

I feel we need to be able to risk some controversy in order to give you some basic concepts and some clear descriptions and contrasts, so that you can further educate yourself about the condition, and possibly start to take a more active role in your treatment. Over the past several years, I have seen that the more patients and their families can learn about their disorder from reliable sources, and the more they can become active participants in their treatment, the better their outcome is likely to be.

Up to now bipolar disorder may have largely felt like a complicated mystery to you, perhaps something like the first quote mentioned at the start of the chapter, from a recent journal article:

"Bipolar disorder (BD) holds the dubious distinction of being one of the most complex conditions faced in psychiatric practice."[2]

It turns out that bipolar disorder and the formulas for successful treatment are much simpler and more straightforward than you might have thought, much more like the second quote mentioned above, at the start of the chapter, from one of my patients:

"Simplicity is the key to complexity."[3]

My goal in this book is to explain these things to you in terms and descriptions which will make them understandable.

It is my sincere hope and intention that this will start to help you unravel the mystery of bipolar disorder, so that you can realistically start to expect and achieve a good outcome.

At the back of the book you will find a Glossary, with a number of terms that will be used repeatedly throughout the book, and an Appendix, with symptom descriptions of the mood disorders from the current diagnostic manual. Understanding these few terms, and/or knowing where to find their definitions if you forget, will help you on your journey through the book.

Chapter 2

Three Important Clinical Research Studies

(Please note: If for any reason you find this chapter or Chapter 3 too academic, simply jump ahead to Chapter 4.)

In the prior chapter I explained to you that bipolar disorder is a very treatable disorder. Unfortunately, despite seeing dedicated and extensively trained health care providers, the majority of bipolar patients in the United States experience only fair to poor outcomes. These outcomes need to be seen as compared to the goal of better functioning as part of stable long-term recovery. This difference between treatability and observed outcomes must leave us all scratching our heads.

You will note that I said "in the United States," and you may be wondering whether it is any different anywhere else in the developed world, and we'll come back to that question later.

To explain the situation in the United States, however, I must first give you some brief background on the clinical research into bipolar disorder treatment. There are two large highly respected multi-university research groups that have done the lion's share of clinical studies of bipolar disorder over the past several years. The first of these is the Stanley Foundation Bipolar Network, or SFBN. Leaders of this group include Robert Post, M.D., Lori Altshuler, M.D., and others. A few years ago this group changed its name to the Bipolar Collaborative Network, or BCN. I will therefore abbreviate this group as SFBN/BCN[c].

Bipolar depression has been felt for quite some time to be one of the biggest unsolved challenges in bipolar disorder treatment,[161,162] so the SFBN/BCN group has studied how we might treat bipolar depression more successfully.

Some earlier studies had shown depression continuing in some patients after treatment with mood stabilizers. The majority of bipolar specialists, including the SFBN/BCN group, has always, based on the scientific evidence, viewed traditional mood stabilizers, specifically lithium, divalproex (Depakote), carbamazepine (Equetro, Tegretol, etc.), and more recently lamotrigine (Lamictal), to be the most effective medication treatments for bipolar disorder. The SFBN/BCN studies have looked at what would happen in bipolar patients suffering with bipolar depression.

One of the three studies emphasized in this chapter started with patients with bipolar depression already being treated with one or more traditional mood stabilizers (abbreviated MSs). The researchers then added an antidepressant medication. The antidepressant was then continued (along with the mood stabilizer[s]) for up to a year, and the researchers observed and recorded the results. I'll abbreviate this first study as Altshuler 1 (2003).[10]

If you ask a clinician who uses antidepressants (abbreviated ADs) in the majority of his or her bipolar patients over the long term (and this appears to be the majority of US clinicians treating bipolar disorder[8,9]), the study they are most likely to mention as providing research documentation and support for this practice is Altshuler 1.[10]

To paraphrase the clinical approach of these clinicians, they seem to reason as follows, "Altshuler 1 shows that the bipolar patients who continued on ADs along with the mood stabilizers did better than those in whom ADs were stopped (and who were then continued on the mood stabilizers alone). Therefore I have concluded that I will maintain most or all of my bipolar patients on ADs for the long haul. Antidepressants seem to help, and I don't notice them causing any

---

c The other large multi-university clinical research group doing large-scale studies of bipolar disorder is the STEP-BD, which began a few years after the SFBN/BCN. This is described a few pages later and in the glossary.

problem. I therefore see no reason to stop them or leave them out of the patient's treatment regimen. They can only help, and to remove the AD would leave the patient vulnerable to depression."

This reading of Alshuler 1 leaves out a few things. First, Dr. Althsuler's SFBN/BCN group looked only at patients with bipolar depression,[11,24] not at all bipolar patients.[10] Patients in manic or mixed episodes of bipolar disorder would be expected to do worse on ADs than depressed bipolar patients.[12,13]

Even starting with only bipolar patients in the depressed phase, however, only about 1 in 6 (15.3%) of these patients made it through the first 2 months on an AD without problems and had a positive response to the AD.[14] The small minority of patients who did well with the addition of the AD seemed to do better staying on it over the course of the next year.[10,15]

In a review article from the same group, they pointed out that, "In the Altshuler et al. studies, those who remained well on any antidepressant for more than 2 months" ... was ... "only 15-20% of those initially treated."[16] A subsequent review by the same group, Post, Altshuler, Frye, and others in 2010 again noted only a "15%" to "16%" rate of sustained response to the addition of an antidepressant medicine in ongoing treatment,[17] again, very consistently, 1 in 6 bipolar patients in the depressed phase.[11] And this is just looking at the SFBN/BCN studies.

The other large multi-university clinical research group, the STEP-BD, also looked at the treatment of bipolar depression by adding ADs to mood stabilizers. Overall, the STEP-BD studies show even less benefit of AD use in depressed bipolar patients than that shown in the SFBN/BCN studies.[18,19] One of the studies, a carefully designed, prospective, randomized study of adding ADs to mood stabilizers for bipolar depression, showed no benefit whatsoever of adding ADs, as compared to adding placebo.[18] A group of senior STEP-BD investigators summarized the results of the numerous STEP-BD studies as follows: "The findings from these studies brought into question the widely practiced use of antidepressants in bipolar depression ..."[204]

As always, there are some methodological issues with clinical research studies.[129] The SFBN/BCN Altshuler 1 study was an "observational" study, that is, patients were not randomized into the two treatment groups, raising the possibility of bias in terms of who went into which treatment group. Nonetheless, Altshuler 1, and the later, randomized SFBN/BCN Altshuler 2 study,[15] raise the strong possibility that about 1 in 6 bipolar depressed patients may do better continuing on the added AD for up to one year, especially if they had a very good and complete initial treatment response for more than just a few weeks.

In my own practice, I am constantly on the lookout for these 1 in 6 patients who may do much better when maintained on ADs for the long term, and when I am convinced I have found them, I definitely continue them on the ADs as part of their ongoing treatment regimen.

It is then interesting to compare the demonstration of effectiveness of adding ADs to core mood stabilizers in just 1 in 6 depressed bipolar patients, with the practice in the United States of prescribing ADs long term to 4 out of 6 of all bipolar patients.[8,9,64]

The SFBN/BCN research group found that the ADs were only successful in 1 in 6 of the bipolar depressed patients in their studies. You might wonder then, whether they found any other medicines or groups of medicines that were successful more often?

It turns out that the SFBN/BCN research group did look at this question in a second important study, a multi-year study of 525 bipolar patients published in late 2010.[20] They found that success rates were higher for lithium, thyroid medicine, anticonvulsants (seizure-reducing medicines, including the anticonvulsant mood stabilizers), the newer antipsychotics (the "atypical" antipsychotics, see Glossary), and even the benzodiazepines (see Glossary). The antidepressants as a class had the 6th-highest success rates. Only the stimulants and the older antipsychotics had lower success rates (see the tables at the end of Chapter 9).[20]

To bring the story full circle, I pointed out that we have only fair to poor clinical outcomes for bipolar patients "in the United States." We must all wonder whether it is any different anywhere else in the developed world. Very interestingly, in the third major study mentioned in the title for this chapter, it was the very same SFBN/BCN group whose studies are held up as a justification for widespread long-term AD use, who recently published a study which addressed this question, Post, Leverich, Altshuler, et al. (2011).[21] They compared the practices and clinical outcomes in the United States with those in two European countries.

They found some surprising differences between prescribing patterns in the US as versus the European countries, as well as differences in clinical outcomes between the two groups. "Lithium was used more frequently in Europe than in the US and had a higher rate of success."[21] "Antidepressants were used more in the US, but had extremely low success rates."[21]

Why on earth then are we prescribing them so much in the US, to 4 out of 6 patients long-term?[8,9] To start to understand why, we turn in the next chapter to a closer look at the two major treatment approaches to bipolar disorder.

Chapter 3

The Two Widely-Used Bipolar Disorder Treatment Strategies

I've been caring for patients as a psychiatrist for 30 years, and I'm a clinical bipolar disorder specialist. The key word here is clinical, as the majority of bipolar specialists are primarily researchers. I have, during the course of my career participated in a small amount of clinical research, but the vast majority of my time has been spent in direct patient care, and most of it seeing patients with mood disorders. About two-thirds of the patients I see now suffer with bipolar disorder, and most of the others suffer with depression.

As my fellow clinical bipolar specialist, Jim Phelps, M.D., recently pointed out,[22,23] the root word for doctor means "teacher." Over the past 20 years focusing on the mood disorders, I have also discovered that a major part of my job is to help patients and their families become experts about their illness, and that this will dramatically improve their outcomes.

There currently seem to be two treatment approaches for bipolar disorder (Table 1), and one of the main goals of this book is to explain them to you. The first approach focuses on the lifetime course of bipolar disorder, including also its patterns of cycling. This cycling is often not just up (mania) or down (depression). The cycling is instead often up and down at the same time to varying degrees (so-called mixed states or mixed episodes, see Glossary), especially after a few years and/or episodes of illness, as described in Chapters 4 and 5.

15

Table 3.1

The Two Common Bipolar Disorder Treatment Strategies		
	CRBBT Cycling and Recurrence-Based Bipolar Treatment	**PBBT** (the most widely used strategy) Polarity-Based Bipolar Treatment
Clinician's View of the Illness	Long-Term/Longitudinal[33,43,143,190]	Short-Term/Cross-Sectional
Markers/ Indicators	Family history, age of onset, lifetime illness course, response to prior treatments, current symptoms	Current symptoms
Primary Phenomena[30]	Cycling and recurrence (up and down *and* mixed episodes)[44]	Manic vs. depressed states (up or down only)[44]
This Approach Fully Explains	**Early** *and* **Late Course** Symptom Patterns[44,89]	**Early Course** symptom Patterns Only[44,89]
Overall Goal	Calm and Dampen Long-Term Cycling[4,5,6,7,43]	Reverse Short-Term Polarity[8,9]
First Treatment Goal	Control Manic and Mixed Symptoms "Mania First"[33,43,152]	Fix Depression[8,9,121,207] "Depression First"
Main Medicines Used	Mood Stabilizers[4-7,33,43,108]	Antidepressants[8,9,121]
Overall Medicines Used	MS>AAP>>AD	AD>AAP>>MS
Antidepressant Use	Infrequent, very selective, sometimes short-term, and usually after better-proven strategies have been exhausted[4,5,6,7]	In the majority of cases[8,9], frequently starting on Day 1[8,9] and long-term[8,9], often uninterrupted for years
Size Of Medication Combinations	Small[41]	Large[41]
Observed Effectiveness	Moderate[20,21]	Extremely low [10,16,19,20,21,28,29,39,42]

MS = *Mood Stabilizers* **AAP** = *Atypical Anti-Psychotics* **AD** = *Anti-Depressants*

The first approach (**cycling and recurrence**) looks closely at patterns of recurrence, that is, how often and under what conditions the patient experiences additional episodes of illness. This approach also focuses somewhat more on manic and mixed episodes, due to the awareness that the frequency and severity of cycling and recurrence cannot be controlled without doing so.

The second approach (**polarity**) is less concerned with the long sweep of the illness over time, and instead focuses on polarity, that is, whether the current episode of illness is up (manic) or down (depressed). The polarity-based approach is tightly linked with the current official diagnostic classification, as contained in the DSM-IV-TR[24] and DSM-IV,[11] which are very similar to one another. Mixed episodes are not felt to occur very often in the view of the polarity model, and these are very narrowly defined[11,24] and therefore less frequently observed in this view.

Practitioners of the polarity approach are much more concerned with depressive symptoms, and seem to find them in a very high proportion of bipolar patients. Please note that the bipolar patients themselves usually don't report mania or manic symptoms on their own in the office.[69,94] They almost always complain instead of what they describe as "depression," almost regardless of their actual mood state. (See the more complete descriptions of this pattern in Chapters 5 and 16.)

The polarity-based practitioners then treat the vast majority of bipolar patients with antidepressants,[8,9,64,208] often from the first day they see them, and then often extending forever after, with occasional or frequent switches of which AD or ADs they are using, but without ever stopping antidepressants altogether, as practitioners working with the polarity approach seem to believe the ADs to be helpful for the majority of patients in both the short term and the long term. Sometimes the ADs are used together with mood stabilizers, and sometimes not.

These practitioners then often explain the long-term use of ADs after the fact with the observation that their patients remain depressed, and are essentially always depressed, and this does seem to be the case; but there is increasing evidence that patients may remain ill because of continued AD use,[12,23,25,26,27,209] rather than in spite of it. (See the interesting discussion of this in the Phelps book,[23] pages 176 to 184.) As noted in Chapter 2, AD use beyond 3 months has been demonstrated to be effective in only 1 in 6 bipolar depressed patients,[16,18,19,21,28-30] so that calling these medicines "antidepressants" when they're being used in the treatment of bipolar disorder is usually not an accurate or reliable description.[28,61,145]

The reason for explaining the two different treatment approaches to you is that the treatment approach used for about two-thirds of bipolar patients in the United States,[8,9,64] is the depression-first polarity view relying most heavily on ADs. Note that AD use has been shown repeatedly by the best available research to lead to

17

"extremely low success rates."[31] [16,18-21,28-30,145]

That is, the polarity-based treatment approach used for the vast majority of bipolar patients in the United States for the past 10 years has repeatedly and consistently been demonstrated to fail in 5 bipolar patients out of 6. Put another way, this strategy fails in bipolar disorder five times as often as it succeeds.

Given the high failure rate, it would seem that polarity-based clinicians aren't generally in a position to expect complete clearing of major mood episodes. They seem to consider the treatment to be as successful as it can be, even if it just succeeds in keeping patients out of hospital, and even if it takes continuing 4 to 8 medicines to do so. These medicines are continued, even though they are often associated with bothersome side effects, including considerable drowsiness, interfering with the patient's ability to function well.

Clinical Case 3.1[14, d]

An obviously disabled 53-year-old man was recently seen for initial evaluation at a public mental health center. No old records were available, but his concerned and supportive sister, a good historian, accompanied him. He gave, and his sister confirmed, an unequivocal history of bipolar I disorder, with a first admission 20 years earlier for mania, and a total of 6 psychiatric admissions, with 5 of the 6 being at nearby university-affiliated teaching hospitals, with lengthy periods of outpatient follow-up with the hospital psychiatrist. The 6th hospitalization was at a state hospital. His diagnosis was bipolar disorder throughout, and he had been treated with numerous antidepressants and antipsychotics over the years. On specific questioning, both he and his sister denied his ever having been treated with lithium, divalproex sodium, or carbamazepine, but after discussion of the options, they readily consented to a trial of lithium,[14] given without antidepressants.

One of my main reasons for writing this book is to re-acquaint patients, families, and clinicians instead with what is now almost a lost art, the simpler and more effective alternative, the evidence-based 'cycling-and-recurrence' approach.[4-7]

---

d Clinical case reproduced from the Journal of Clinical Psychiatry, 2010, with permission from Physicians Postgraduate Press, Inc.

The cycling-and-recurrence approach has been shown to lead to moderate success rates,[20,21] and in my experience with the strategies described in this book, can lead to moderate to high success rates in clinical practice. The goal of the cycling-and-recurrence based approach is much more ambitious as compared to the very limited improvement generally possible with the polarity-based approach, as you'll see later in the chapter.

About 12 years ago I read what turned out to be a very important article[31] on the treatment of bipolar disorder. The article got me started thinking about the above two approaches, and I started more carefully watching and contrasting the 2 approaches in my work with my own patients and those of others. I found that the 'cycling-and-recurrence' approach described in this article[31] consistently led to better patient outcomes, and so I began studying this approach in even more detail. As others found out about my interest in bipolar disorder, I started seeing more and more bipolar patients.

This approach is described in Table 1 as cycling-and-recurrence-based bipolar treatment, or CRBBT for short. Cycling simply means that the activation[e] and mood state of the bipolar disorder varies up and down, and often both up and down to varying degrees at the same time, with various patterns emerging over the lifetime course of the disorder.

The number of cycling patterns are almost unlimited,[4,169] but some patterns have been better defined and understood, and may have very important meanings as to which treatments might be more successful. Therefore, determining and understanding a patient's pattern of cycling may be very important for the treatment. In CRBBT, for example, there is much more emphasis on the fact that the mood swings may be quite variable, and often mixed (up and down at the same time or within a short span of time), rather than simply up or down. As the most respected text on bipolar disorder, Goodwin and Jamison (2007),[4] states,

"Thus, far from being a 'bipolar' disorder, with the assumption of clinically opposite states, the illness is characterized by co-occurrence of manic and depressive symptoms more often than not."[32]

That is, highs and lows of activation and mood often happen at the same time,

---

e "Activation" simply refers to how energetic or "wound up" a patient is. See also the Glossary at the back of the book, and especially Chapter 16.

rather than at separate times, and this is especially true after a few episodes or a few years of the bipolar disorder, in the late course of bipolar disorder, as described in Chapters 4 and 5.

Recurrence simply refers to the fact that in bipolar disorder, the episodes happen again and again, with varying patterns and frequencies.

CRBBT takes a long-term view of the lifetime history of mood episodes, as this often provides important clues, both to possible progression of the illness over time, and to which treatments might be most successful at the current phase of the illness. CRBBT is much more direct in describing bipolar disorder as a dominant lifelong illness, which is viewed as more important than other disorders, and the primary focus of treatment.

The main exceptions to this rule are if the patient has active alcohol or drug abuse, or a medical or neurologic brain disorder, at the same time as the bipolar disorder. In such cases CRBBT considers both disorders to be very important, and they must both be treated from the beginning. These exceptions are also so-called Top-Tier disorders, and are discussed in some detail in Chapter 12.

The CRBBT view of the illness takes into account family history of bipolar disorder and other mood disorders, age of onset of mood episodes, lifetime history of all mood episodes, and history of responses to prior treatments, as well as the current mood state.[4,5,6,7] In summary, four of the five key factors in the CRBBT view of the illness are historical, or part of the long-term view of the illness,[33] and only one of the five is the current mood state. This is in contrast to the polarity-based approach, which tends to view bipolar disorder primarily as the current mood state.

The initial goal of CRBBT is to control the manic and mixed symptoms,[33,43,152] as these include severe insomnia, irritability, agitation, and inability to think clearly due to racing thoughts and distractibility. They also include impulsive and high risk behavior and increased risk for suicidal thoughts and behavior.[33-35,43,110] These symptoms often lead to unnecessary relationship break-ups, job loss (often due to being disruptive and getting fired), and driving away friends and family. In summary, these patients are at risk of losing just about everything, unless these symptoms are rapidly brought under control. Usually the overall mood cycling is much more easily controlled if these manic and mixed symptoms are controlled at the beginning and kept under control for the duration of the illness.

Successful treatment of these symptoms often leads to a significant reduction in the patient's depressive symptoms as well. If some of the depressive symptoms persist, they can often be successfully addressed after control of the manic and mixed symptoms, as described in Chapter 9.

Less often, in about 15% to 20% of bipolar patient visits in my experience, the patient with known bipolar I or bipolar II disorder may present with a pure bipolar depression, with markedly excessive sleep (11 to 20 hours per 24 hours), and extreme reduction in energy, interest, and activity. This treatment situation is specifically addressed in Chapter 9. In such cases, the depression must be addressed immediately, and this includes starting mood stabilizer treatment at the beginning, to protect against increased mood cycling, as well as potential swings into manic or mixed states.

The medium- to long-term goal of CRBBT is to control and smooth out the mood cycling, and also to reduce the frequency of later episodes. As I explain it to my patients, we want to compress the range of swings to the center, and spread out the frequency of episodes, as shown in the following graphic by the shift from pattern A to pattern B:

Figure 3.1

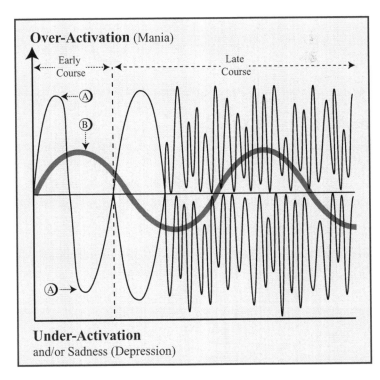

21

The long term goal of CRBBT is to smooth the cycling to such a degree that we prevent full mood episodes altogether, and thereby make it possible for the patient to develop more complete recovery of functioning in all areas of their lives.

The main medications used in CRBBT are the traditional mood stabilizers (MSs), lithium, divalproex (Depakote), carbamazepine (Equetro, Tegretol, and others), and lamotrigine (lamotrigine). We sometimes prescribe 2 or 3 of them at a time, if needed, with or without the newer antipsychotics, which are commonly referred to as the Atypical AntiPsychotics (AAPs). The atypical antipsychotics, as well as lithium, divalproex, and carbamazepine, are all effective against manic and mixed symptoms. The three original well-established traditional mood stabilizers (lithium, divalproex/Depakote, and carbamazepine) have been used successfully for decades and proven in hundreds of studies. They have powerful anti-manic effects, and are thus described in more detail in Chapter 8 as **ceilings**, that is, they control or prevent excessive "up" swings.

The newest traditional mood stabilizer, lamotrigine (Lamictal), is not especially good for manic symptoms, and is only mildly helpful for acute depression, but it is much more powerful in protecting against the return of depressive episodes, and is therefore described in Chapter 8 as a **floor**, that is, protects against excessive "down" swings.[36] Lithium has some of this effect as well. All four of the mood stabilizers provide some degree of smoothing and reducing the frequency of cycling over time, and I refer to this as **core** stabilization.

In the CRBBT approach, there is concern that the antidepressant (AD) medications may trigger manic or mixed episodes in some patients,[37] worse mixed episodes,[13,131] and increased frequency of mood cycles, so-called rapid cycling.[19,27] They have also been associated with more frequent and worse depressions,[12,23,25,26] and more suicidal behaviors in bipolar patients.[38]

As a result CRBBT-oriented clinicians don't usually use antidepressants early on in the treatment process, and we use them very selectively, as for example possibly in the approximately 15% to 20% of bipolar patients who present with pure bipolar depression. We may also use them short-term, i.e., for just 2-3 months, and even then often after a trial of the better-proven olanzapine-fluoxetine combination.[102,128,131]

Aside from the infrequent patients with pure bipolar depression, we usually use antidepressant medicines only after the numerous better-proven strategies[4,5,6,7,20,21,131,187] described in Chapters 8 and 9 have been exhausted. So, for instance, a clinician using the CRBTT approach might consider antidepressant medicines 4th, 5th, or 6th in the process of building a regimen, if at all, and only when combined with mood stabilizers.

Clinicians working with the more commonly used polarity-based treatment approach are generally using antidepressants instead as the 1st or 2nd medicine tried, often without mood stabilizers, and then sometimes continuing the antidepressants forever without interruption, despite strong evidence that they fail in 5 patients out of 6, and are actually more likely to make things worse rather than better over the long term.[12,25,26,39,40,131,186,209]

The eventual size of the treatment regimen needed to treat bipolar disorder with CRBBT is usually relatively smaller,[41] i.e., fewer medicines are needed. This may perhaps be because the mood stabilizers have been shown to be more effective than the antidepressants[18,19,20,21] in bipolar I and II disorder. (For the diagnostic manual description of bipolar I and II disorder, see the Appendix.[24])

The long-term success rates of the CRBBT approach as demonstrated in systematic studies are moderate,[20,111,116,187] and I believe from my own experience, and using strategies outlined in this book, that this approach can have moderate to high success rates when applied in clinical practice.

We'll now look at further differences between CRBBT and the more popular strategy used in about two-thirds of patients in the United States,[8,9,64] described here as polarity-based bipolar treatment, or PRBBT (See Table 1).

In polarity-based treatment, the antidepressants are often paired with a newer/"atypical" antipsychotic. More recently, the antidepressants are increasingly paired with lamotrigine (Lamictal), which unfortunately provides only weak anti-manic effects.

Many clinicians using the polarity-based approach don't view bipolar disorder as such a dominant illness (See also Chapter 12), but perhaps more as one illness or condition among many that a patient may have all at the same time.

As a result, various symptom clusters that show up in the patient are often felt by polarity-based clinicians to be separate and equally important disorders,[106] rather than expressions of the primary bipolar disorder. Some examples include insomnia, anxiety, obsessions, depression, poor concentration, lack of energy, and irritability.

Often, various medications are added to address these seeming surface complaints as if they were separate conditions, without a careful look at the state of the underlying mood cycling. So, for instance, many patients end up with the addition of anti-anxiety medications for reported anxiety, an antidepressant for depression, a sleep medication for the insomnia, and stimulants for treatment of presumed co-occurring ADHD (attention-deficit hyperactivity disorder).[219] As described in Chapter 12, all these different symptom patterns can easily be mimicked by mania or mixed states, which may then go untreated or under-treated.

As you can see (also in Chapter 15), the medication regimens tend to get large,[41] sometimes with a medication for every symptom cluster, but with a failure to evaluate and successfully treat the underlying bipolar disorder, which is often generating most or all these symptoms.

The bottom line, though, would appear to be long-term effectiveness. As noted in Chapter 2, antidepressant medicines are used more often by polarity-based clinicians than the traditional mood stabilizers, but the antidepressant use is associated with "extremely low success rates."[21]

Why then, would two out of three US bipolar patients[8,9,92,131] be treated with them?

To start figuring this out, we need to start looking in the next chapter at how bipolar disorder develops over time.

Chapter 4

The Natural Life History of Bipolar Disorder

As little as thirty to thirty-five years ago, many psychiatrists felt that bipolar disorder was unlikely to occur in children. This view shifted only gradually until about the last fifteen years, during which time it has shifted dramatically and controversially with emerging studies.

With a rapid increase in rates of diagnosing bipolar disorder in children,[50] there are understandable concerns that childhood bipolar disorder might be overdiagnosed.[51,52]

At the same time, Ellen Leibenluft, M.D., at the National Institutes of Mental Health (NIMH) has reported a different and previously unrecognized disorder with continuous irritability, rather than episodes of irritability, called severe mood dysregulation (SMD),[53,181] which may include a number of the children recently diagnosed as having bipolar disorder.

Other conditions may, of course, have some symptoms similar to those of bipolar disorder, such as ADHD, drug abuse, childhood trauma, chaotic home, etc., and the clinician has to distinguish very carefully among these somewhat similar and often overlapping symptomatic conditions before deciding on the primary diagnosis.

On the other hand, a number of studies show that a large proportion of bipolar patients, perhaps as many as half, has onset of mood episodes by age nineteen.[54,130] There is also evidence that successive groups of patients born in later decades (for instance those born in the 1970s compared to those born in the 1950s) are experiencing mood symptoms beginning at earlier and earlier ages.[54]

Bipolar patients tend to experience their first depressive episode earlier than patients with major depressive disorder.[62,146,158] In one study the bipolar patients had their first depressive episode at an average age of 21, whereas patients with major depressive disorder had their first mood episode at an average age of 30.[158] A first major depressive episode before age 25 may actually be a clue that the patient's primary diagnosis is bipolar disorder rather than major depressive disorder,[159] as may 2 or more failed trials of antidepressants.[180,182,200]

There are three different severity grades of bipolar disorder. Bipolar I disorder has longer, more severe episodes, and causes significant life disruption. Bipolar II disorder has shorter episodes of moderate severity, but may cause just as much overall life disruption as bipolar I disorder. Bipolar disorder NOS (bipolar disorder not otherwise specified) has overall less severe episodes and a much more vaguely defined clinical picture. More complete descriptions of these conditions are found in the Glossary, and specific DSM-IV-TR criteria[24] are described in the Appendix. If one includes all three severity grades of bipolar disorder, the overall lifetime occurrence of bipolar disorder is in the 3% to 4% range.[1,45,55]

Recently, a German and Swiss research study followed a large group of depressed patients out over 10 years. They had originally been diagnosed with unipolar depression (major depressive disorder,[24] that is regular depression, without any episodes of mania, mixed state, or minor mania [hypomania], ever). However, as the patients were observed and evaluated over time, about 40% of them were found to have disorders that were actually discovered to be in the range of bipolar disorders, instead of depression only.[55] An earlier French study found that more in-depth evaluation of major depression patients showed that 40% of them actually had bipolar spectrum disorders (see Glossary) instead of major depression.[146]

To summarize, we now view bipolar disorder as a more common disorder with a broader range of symptom pictures, and an earlier age of onset. Also, if we evaluate more carefully and over time, what initially looks like major depressive disorder may actually turn out, in many patients, to be bipolar disorder instead.

Bipolar disorder follows a somewhat predictable progression (worsening over time),[57,58] but this progression is frequently and sometimes dramatically accelerated by a number of factors, including childhood onset.

Early course and late course bipolar disorder have such different symptom patterns that one could easily be fooled into thinking that they were different disorders altogether, rather than the expectable change in symptoms of bipolar disorder over time. Clinicians (and also patients and families) must therefore be familiar with the general pattern of progression of bipolar disorder. This will help them recognize the condition as bipolar disorder in the first place, and also help them estimate where the patient's current state fits on the progression.

At this point we'll start explaining the symptoms seen in the **early course** of the life history of bipolar disorder. Some patients describe chronic inability to sleep, often beginning in childhood,[56,203] and sometimes before other symptoms of illness appear.

Once the mood episodes themselves begin, the early life history of the bipolar disorder (early course) often lasts for the first five to ten years of illness, or the first five episodes.[57,58] If, however, the bipolar disorder begins in childhood, half or more of these patients seem to skip the early course altogether and start immediately with late course symptoms.[87,88]

Early course bipolar disorder symptoms include simple depressive, manic, or hypomanic (small manic) episodes (with the shorthand for these being D, M, m, respectively). Simple sequences of episodes are also common at this stage, for example MDi (**M**anic, then **D**epressed, then well **i**nterval), DMi (**D**epressed, then **M**anic, then well **i**nterval), and MDMD (**M**anic – > **D**epressed – > **M**anic – >**D**epressed). The specific patterns are of some importance; for instance the MDi pattern is associated with a higher likelihood of a good response to lithium.[157]

Bipolar disorder is easier to treat during the early course.[57,58] Many patients respond well to treatment with a single medicine, such as lithium or other traditional mood stabilizers (MSs), such as divalproex (Depakote), carbamazepine (Equetro, Tegretol, and others), or lamotrigine (Lamictal), so long as these are given in the absence of antidepressants.

Unfortunately, a 2007 study on the course of bipolar disorder found, "The time span between onset of illness and initiation of psychiatric care was on average nearly 4 years, and time between onset and start of MSs was more than 14 years. Medication with MSs substantially decreased the frequency of episodes."[58]

In other words, even though MSs were found to be very helpful in decreasing the frequency of episodes, patients had a delay of 14 years before they received them. This finding of a long delay (of 5 to even 16 years) from onset of illness to diagnosis of bipolar disorder and the start of mood stabilizer treatment has also been found in numerous other studies.[31,58,63-66,146,156,159,172,173,201,202,211]

You might wonder what is prescribed instead of MSs. Two large pharmacy data base studies of bipolar patients found that the most frequently prescribed medicines were not the MSs, but the antidepressants (ADs).[8,9]

Unfortunately, the ADs fail to provide any benefit beyond 3 months of treatment in 5 out of 6 bipolar patients,[10,14,16,18,21,28,29,38,42,114] even those selected as being in the midst of bipolar depression. As one recent review summarized, "The treatment of bipolar depression differs from that of recurrent major depression in that the efficacy of conventional antidepressant drugs is not well-established."[135]

That is, the "ADs"[28,145] work pretty well for many patients with major depressive disorder,[26] but they don't work for the vast majority of bipolar patients.[131,174,182] Since they seem to work for unipolar (major depressive disorder) patients but not for bipolar patients, they might be more accurately described as "unipolar antidepressants."[28,61] Alternatively, when used in bipolar patients, they might be called "1-chance-in-6 antidepressants," because that is about how often they work.

The conventional/unipolar ADs are also associated with worsening of rapid cycling[12,19,27,131,186] and worsening of mixed episodes.[11,131] In what may come as a surprise to almost everyone, ADs are also associated with worse and more frequent bipolar depressive episodes.[12,25,26]

For instance, a multi-center European study of 2,416 adult bipolar patients evaluated in the manic phase of bipolar disorder found that those on ADs were significantly more likely to have "mixed episodes, anxiety, or rapid cycling, and have a higher risk of depression during follow-up" than those not on antidepressants.[12] That is, those on ADs were more likely to have developed the symptoms of more advanced or late course bipolar disorder than those not on ADs,[21,186] including more depression.[161,162]

Patients who have been subjected to a larger number of AD medication treatment trials have also been found to have more suicidal thoughts and behaviors[38,59] and more likelihood of failure to respond to subsequent treatments.[60]

"Antidepressant" medicines (unipolar ADs) may also cause the failure of mood stabilizer trials. That is, the same mood stabilizers may be considerably more effective in different treatment trials without the ADs.[170]

In summary, the ADs seem to be associated with the appearance of more and more unstable mood states in bipolar patients. Antidepressants appear to be linked to worse and faster mood cycles[186] and the progression of bipolar illness,[21] and also, surprisingly enough, to worse depression and suicidal behaviors.

As you might have already suspected, late course bipolar patients have more complex and at times more severe episodes of mood disorder, with a somewhat more depressive[161,162] and "mixed" flavor (manic and depressive symptoms occurring at the same time),[131] with briefer pauses between illness episodes,[58] and with more rapid cycling, ultra-rapid, and ultradian cycling,[21] worse anxiety,[12] and some with "highly recurrent refractory depression"[179] as part of the rapid cycling.

From the previous discussion, you will also note that these are exactly the patterns with which use of the ADs are associated. Interestingly, the 2010 study by Post, Altshuler, Leverich, et al., previously mentioned in Chapter 2 found much more AD use in the US, and more complex and severe late course symptoms like those above in the patients in the US, when compared with treatments and patients' bipolar illnesses in the Netherlands and Germany,[21] who tended to have more successful treatments and less severe bipolar illnesses. Is this all a coincidence? We don't really know yet, but there seem to be enough coincidences to raise at least a tiny bit of suspicion.

In order to make the diagnosis of bipolar disorder at all, the clinicians using the polarity-based view of bipolar disorder (described in Chapter 3) need to find clear current or recent manic episodes, but pure manias are considerably less frequent in the late course of bipolar disorder. That is, the current standard diagnostic manual, the DSM-IV-TR,[24] describes the early course bipolar features fairly well, but by the time the patient gets to treatment, they are in the late course of bipolar disorder,[21] and the DSM-IV-TR categories aren't very useful at all by then.

Because of the previously described 5 to 16 year delay in diagnosis, a high proportion of patients are already in the late course of bipolar disorder by the time they are diagnosed. If the patient happens to see a clinician who operates from the polarity-based view of bipolar disorder and relies on the polarity-based criteria of the DSM-IV-TR,[24] the clinician is then looking for current or very recent pure manic episodes, which are often no longer there in the late course. The polarity-based clinician may therefore conclude that the patient has major depressive disorder, rather than bipolar disorder. This then often leads to the diagnosis of bipolar disorder being missed during the late course.

I have also repeatedly seen instances where a first clinician, we'll call her clinician A, treated the patient during a manic episode, and therefore made the diagnosis of bipolar disorder. Then eventually the patient would see a second clinician, clinician B, a few years later. Clinician B, operating from the polarity-based view, would note the relative *current* absence of pure manias at the time when he was seeing the patient, without taking an adequate history of the patient's lifetime course of mood symptoms, or perhaps disbelieving or dismissing this earlier history of manic episode for whatever reason.

This would then lead clinician B to mistakenly change the previous diagnosis of bipolar disorder made by clinician A, to a diagnosis of major depressive disorder.[11,24] Clinician B would then change the treatment to one intended to treat major depressive disorder, and the patient's condition would then get worse.

The patient would then later come to me, and when I did review the lifetime history of mood episodes, I would find out that the patient had indeed suffered manic episodes at some point (often during the early course of the disorder). This would then indicate that clinician A's original diagnosis of bipolar disorder was indeed correct. (Note that if one has an accurate diagnosis of a manic or mixed or hypomanic episode at any point in one's life, the diagnosis remains bipolar disorder ever after, and never, ever changes back to major depressive disorder.) When I would then switch the patient's medicines from those for major depressive disorder to those more appropriate for bipolar disorder, the patient would improve a great deal, and stay significantly better for months to years.

In the late course of bipolar disorder, when a careful history of mood symptoms is taken, **mixed episodes** are perhaps the most common symptom pattern.[4,72,77,78,131] Repeated, more frequent, and at times seemingly untreatable depressions appear commonly,[179] although if one asks very carefully, and also has the observations of a key support person either present in the session, or contacted during the session with the patient's permission, one finds in my experience that the majority of these episodes are not pure bipolar depressive episodes, but rather mixed episodes.

Mixed episodes appear, along with the development of **rapid cycling** (and **ultra-rapid** and **ultradian cycling**,[188,189] see below), to be the standard features of the bipolar disorder late course.[21] The DSM-IV-TR[24] definition of **rapid cycling** involves four or more illness episodes per year, with episodes followed either by a shift into the opposite polarity (that is mania to depression, or depression to mania), or 2 months of partial or complete symptom clearing between episodes. Rapid cycling is represented schematically in Figure 4.1 below.

Figure 4.1

Rapid Cycling

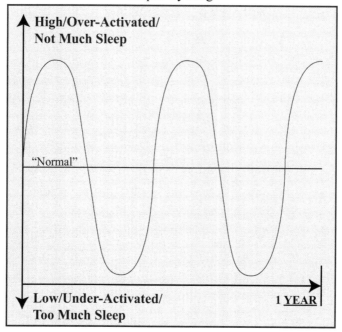

Many patients in the late course experience cycling much more rapid than rapid cycling, such as **ultra-rapid cycling**, that is, multiple distinct mood episodes within a week[5,188,189] (Figure 4.2 below),

Figure 4.2

Ultra-Rapid Cycling

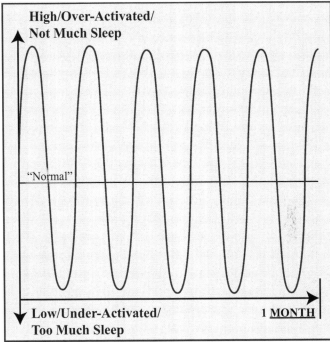

or even **ultradian cycling**, which is multiple mood episodes within the same day.[4,6,188,189] (Figure 4.3 below).

Figure 4.3

Ultradian Cycling

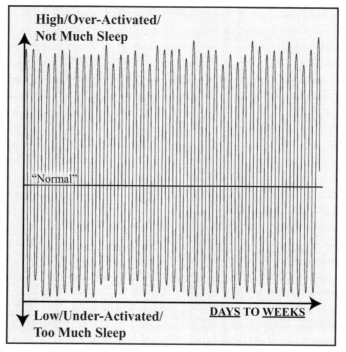

Note that in Figures 4.1, 4.2, and 4.3 above, the cycling is represented schematically as having artificially regular, predictable, and equal cycles, up and then down, and then up again, etc. The actual cycling patterns of real patients' bipolar illnesses, however, are just as often irregular, unpredictable, and unequal, that is, totally chaotic and unpredictable high and low swings, something like Figure 4.4 below, or Figure 5.2 in the next chapter, but often a lot more irregular and unpredictable than these.

In my work as a bipolar specialist, most of the patients I see have had years of bipolar illness, years of diagnostic delay, and years of previous treatments. The vast majority of these patients are therefore well into the late course of bipolar disorder.

At the time of their first visit with me about half of them already have ultra-rapid or ultradian cycling. The cycling for this group is measured less in number of episodes per year (as it is in rapid cycling), and more nearly in number of episodes per week, or per day. Their cycling seems to be more nearly 'rabid' than 'rapid'.

In the process of asking their manic and depressive symptoms in considerable detail, I have found that a more accurate explanation of these patients' ultra-rapid or ultradian cycling would be to view it as a mix of rapidly shifting manic and depressive symptoms.[4,77] This is then often basically a single ongoing, extremely **rapidly shifting mixed episode**[189] (RSME, Figure 4.4 below).

Fig 4.4

Rapidly Shifting

Mixed Episode (RSME)

Please note: The actual mood cycling of bipolar patients is often much more irregular, complex, and unpredictable than this simplified illustration.

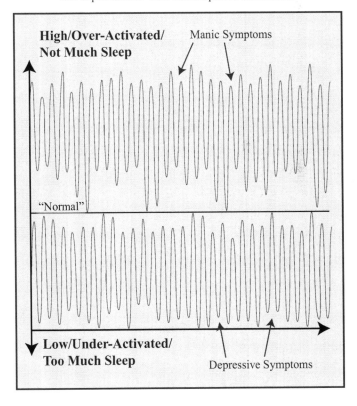

Please note that my description of mixed episodes is somewhat broader than that of DSM-IV-TR,[11,24] and I'll explain the difference and its importance in the next chapter. Mixed episodes are so important to the understanding of the late course of bipolar disorder that they are the subject of the entire next chapter (Chapter 5).

Unipolar "antidepressants" started or continued during these mixed episodes masquerading as bipolar "depression" are generally not helpful, and may maintain or worsen the mixed states[13,68,72,131] and possibly even the depression itself.[12,25,26] Note that not a single antidepressant is FDA (Food and Drug Administration) approved for the treatment of bipolar depression or mixed states, and that even the combination of the newer antipsychotic olanzapine (Zyprexa) and the antidepressant fluoxetine (Prozac) (Olanzapine-Fluoxetine Combination, "OFC," trade name Symbyax) is FDA-approved only for bipolar depression, but not for bipolar mixed states.[67]

True pure bipolar depressive episodes are certainly present in the late course, but only in about 15 to 20% of patients in my experience, and almost always associated with a pattern of sleeping extremely long times (i.e., the patient sleeps 10 to 20 hours per 24 hours).[146,154] There may also be additional hours when they lie in bed awake, so as to try to hide from the painful feelings of the depression.

In the past I found myself, almost by reflex, shaving an hour or two off the patient's initial report of the number of hours of sleep, thinking "They can't possibly be sleeping that much!" But then I eventually learned to ask them which specific hours they slept, "From when to when?" Their initial reports in the range of 10 to 20 hours per 24 hours were, to my considerable surprise, confirmed again and again.

It is crucial in this late course phase (as always) to inquire specifically about hours of sleep, irritability, impulsive behavior, racing thoughts, etc., as **bipolar patients almost always emphasize the depressive symptoms instead.**[69,94,131,159] They frequently forget, hesitate to mention, or significantly downplay, the degree and impact of their manic symptoms.

With regard to the racy and over-energetic manic symptoms, the patients generally feel they're just fine, and that everyone else around them must be slowed down and operating in slow motion, or possibly even depressed. Unless the patients themselves feel slowed down or "depressed" in some way or other, they aren't even likely to make or keep an appointment with a clinician.

As a recent article noted, "Because patients with bipolar disorder often do not present in the manic or hypomanic phase of the illness, the presence of these episodes requires a history of these symptoms to be elicited, which may be difficult when patients present during a period of depression."[85] That is, when the patients are manic or hypomanic, they aren't likely to make or keep appointments, so the clinician isn't likely to see them in this state.

The manic, over-energized symptoms are, however, usually quite obvious and often very disruptive to the people closest to the patient. Unless the family or close support person brings the patient in, however, the patient may well just not show up in the clinician's office.

Studies of bipolar patients and clinical observation have repeatedly shown that bipolar patients have distinct thinking problems.[83,84,136] Patients with manic symptoms tend to lack inhibition,[84] and also lack insight,[159] especially into their manic symptoms.

Until the patient is well stabilized, it is therefore extremely valuable to have the patient come to most of their appointments accompanied by a spouse, or by one very close and trusted friend or relative who knows the patient well and sees them on a regular basis. This then substantially increases the likelihood of detecting the manic parts of the illness, which are otherwise easily missed, and which remain important in the late course of bipolar disorder, which is explained further in the next chapter.

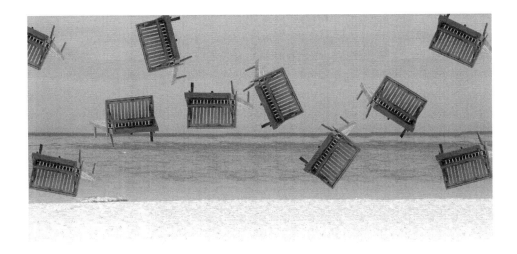

Chapter 5

"All Mixed Up"

The Natural Life History of Bipolar Disorder, Part 2:

The Bipolar Disorder Late Course

In which almost every
patient visit with the psychiatrist begins with the patient complaining of
depression,
but careful evaluation
shows that at least 2/3 of them are actually presenting with mixed episode

"Things are seldom what they seem,
Skim milk masquerades as cream."

Gilbert and Sullivan,
H.M.S. Pinafore

As a result of the factors discussed in Chapter 4, many if not most bipolar patients do not see a psychiatrist until a few years into their disorder. They thus arrive at the psychiatrist in the late course of the bipolar illness. More often than not, they arrive on antidepressant (AD) medications rather than mood stabilizers,[8,9,64,92] or possibly on a combination of ADs and newer antipsychotic medicines, the so-called "atypical antipsychotics" (AAPs). Careful evaluation shows that although the vast majority of these patients complain of being "depressed," they are actually presenting with more broadly defined mixed episodes.[57,69,70,71,72,80,94]

When the patient does come in, one of the problems is that there is rarely time for the health care provider to ask the symptoms in more detail, so the practitioner often doesn't ask about hours of sleep per night, irritability, racing thoughts, distractibility, impulsive behavior, etc., i.e., manic or hypomanic symptoms. These are, however, present in about 2/3 of such bipolar patients complaining of depression.[72]

The DSM-IV-TR[24 f] and its predecessor, the DSM-IV,[11] both state that to qualify as a mixed episode, "The criteria are met both for a Manic Episode… and for a Major Depressive Episode … nearly every day during at least a 1-week period."

Figure 5.1 (DSM-IV-TR Mixed Episode)

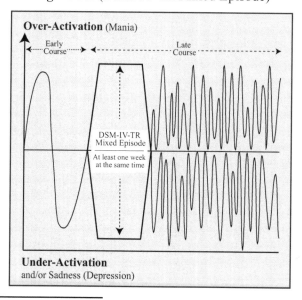

---

f See also DSM-IV-TR diagnostic criteria in Appendix 1 at the back of the book.

These criteria for mixed episode are so narrow and demanding that 5% or fewer of patients coming to a psychiatrist's office will meet these criteria. As the most respected textbook on bipolar disorder asks, "Are the diagnostic criteria of DSM-IV[11] prohibitively strict, as most researchers think?"[73] Put another way, the DSM-IV[11] and DSM-IV-TR[24] rules for diagnosing mixed episode are so strict that very few bipolar disorders play by them.

If one follows these DSM-IV or DSM-IV-TR criteria closely, one thereby ends up labeling about 95% of patients as if they were either simply manic or depressed, as if there were almost no mixed episodes. This DSM-IV-TR[24] description fits pretty well for patients in the early course of bipolar disorder (as described in Chapter 4), because early course patients tend to have somewhat simpler mood episodes than late course patients.

When bipolar disorder begins at or before age 18 (as appears to happen in up to half of all bipolar patients[130]), the illness may shift into the late course of the disorder much more rapidly, sometimes even with the very first mood episodes. That is, many patients with childhood onset of bipolar disorder (in some studies more than half of such patients) seem to skip the simpler early course episodes altogether, and start out immediately with late course illness with mixed episodes and rapid cycling, right from the very beginning.[74,75,76,87,88]

Therefore, by the time patients are being treated by a clinician for bipolar disorder, they are almost all in the late course of the disorder. The DSM-IV-TR[24] description would have us believe that almost all patients are either manic or depressed, with just a very tiny minority suffering with pure mixed episode, as one might expect in early course bipolar disorder.

This description, however, doesn't fit the observed symptom patterns of late course bipolar disorder very well at all. The result is that clinicians are seeing late course bipolar patients,[21] and trying to manage them with a DSM-IV-TR treatment roadmap that describes early course bipolar illness patterns instead. How clinicians and patients are supposed to succeed with this particular setup remains a mystery. This may certainly be one of the factors in the low treatment success rates seen in the US.[20,21,210]

Compare the very narrow description of mixed episode in the DSM-IV-TR[24] with the view of the most highly respected textbook on bipolar disorder,

Goodwin and Jamison (2007),[4] as previously mentioned:

"Finally, although much of the clinical description presented here emphasizes differences among clinical states, we stress from the outset that the coexistence of affective states is fundamental to bipolar disorder and that oscillation into, out of, and within the various forms and states of manic-depressive illness is, in its own right, a hallmark of the disease."[77]

"Thus, far from being a "bipolar" disorder with the assumption of clinically opposite states, the illness is characterized by co-occurrence of manic and depressive symptoms more often than not."[77]

Translation: Bipolar patients' symptoms (especially during the late course) are moving frequently into and out of various degrees of both mania and depression at the same time, most of the time, as shown in Figure 5.2 below.[78]

Figure 5.2

Depression During Mania:
Simultaneous Ratings

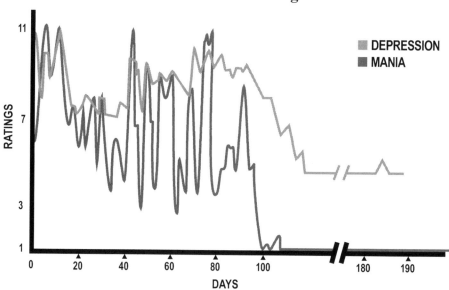

(Source: Kotin J, Goodwin FK, American Journal of Psychiatry 1972, reference 78, reproduced with permission of the American Psychiatric Association.)

Figure 5.2 above shows the charting of both manic and depressive symptoms (shown as dark gray and light gray lines moving above the baseline) in a single patient over a 6-month period.

To summarize the above, there are many more patients (in my experience about 70% of the bipolar patients coming to a psychiatrist's office[72,147]) who fit into more broadly-defined mixed episodes.[69,70,71,72,94,118,171] These are episodes that have a depression or a mania, and at least 2 or 3 symptoms of the opposite "polarity" (direction). It turns out that this broader definition of mixed episode[71,72,79, 80,118] is clinically much more useful than the artificially narrow DSM-IV-TR[24] definition, because it describes the late course bipolar patients we actually see, and helps to guide treatment toward better outcomes.

For instance, there was a recent study by Goldberg and others of patients with a bipolar depressive episode who also had just 2 or more manic symptoms at the same time.[13] Using the broader description of mixed episodes, we would call this "depressive mixed episode," or DMX.[79,80]

DSM-IV-TR,[24] on the other hand, calls this "bipolar depression", rather than mixed episode. In the Goldberg study, adding ADs to mood stabilizers (MSs) did not speed up the time to recovery of these patients. Patients who received the added ADs did, however, have worse manic symptoms (and thereby overall worsening of their condition) at 3 month follow-up compared to those continued on MSs without adding ADs.[13]

Another large multi-center study similarly found that full bipolar depression that also had even "minimal manic symptoms at baseline" was "associated with antidepressant-treatment-emergent mania or hypomania,"[68] that is, manic or hypomanic episodes that began after the addition of ADs. (The symptoms of manic and hypomanic episodes[11,24] are listed in Appendix 1 at the back of the book.)

Translation: If bipolar patients with depression had even a little bit of mania, the mania, and thereby the patient's overall condition, got worse after adding ADs.

In such situations, to call these episodes bipolar depression rather than mixed states, may lead to trouble. To call them "bipolar depression" invites the clinician to think that, because it's "called" bipolar "depression," then it's likely to respond well to adding or continuing "ADs," which these disorders, which are better understood as mixed states, do not.

Yet a third study found that "Even modest manic symptoms during bipolar depressive episodes were associated with greater impulsivity, and with histories of alcohol abuse and suicide attempts."[170]

With the broader definition of mixed episodes, these patients would be described as having depressive mixed episode, DMX.[79,80] This is "a more common, severe, and psychopathologically complex clinical state than pure bipolar depression," so as to "merit recognition as a distinct nosologic entity."[72]

Translation: It's a very common mood state (much more common than pure bipolar depression), but a more complex and severe state, with greater suicide risk,[59,110,118,170] that deserves its own diagnostic label (such as depressive mixed episode, or DMX).

The broader mixed episode definition is thus more helpful, as it identifies the most common late course presentation as mixed episode. It can thereby alert the clinician to the low likelihood of benefit in these patients of adding ADs, and the real possibility of worsening the patient's condition by adding ADs.[13,39,68]

The systematic study of treatments likely to be more successful in DMX is just beginning. The first randomized clinical trial published in 2012[218] showed the AAP ziprasidone (Geodon) to be dramatically superior to placebo in the treatment of acute DMX.

Manic mixed episode (with more manic than depressive symptoms, MMX) is almost as common as DMX in my clinical experience. The very restrictively defined DSM-IV-TR[24] mixed episode (abbreviated here as MIX) is much less common than DMX or MMX. The MIX group must by definition have full and persistent manic symptoms and full and persistent depressive symptoms for a week to qualify for the diagnosis of DSM-IV-TR mixed episode (See Glossary and Appendix). Patients with the MMX or MIX pictures are likely to respond possibly even worse than the DMX group to attempts to treat any depressive symptoms by adding ADs.

If the distribution of patients with the various subtypes of bipolar disorder occurred purely by chance, it might look like Figure 5.3 below:

Figure 5.3

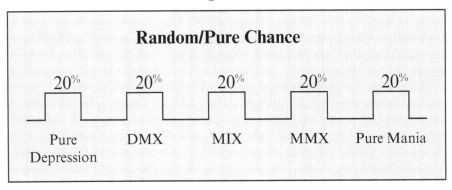

In my experience, what we actually see in the Early Course patients over time is more like this:

Figure 5.4

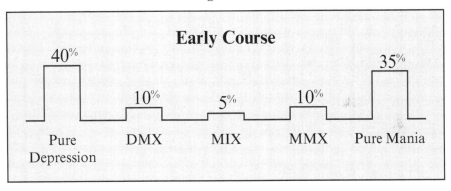

Be aware, of course, that patients' illnesses do not always fit in neat categories. The patients rarely read the books or articles and then control their symptom clusters so as to fit into such neat boxes. In the early course, however, the episodes are generally simpler, cleaner, and closer to fitting in the neat boxes.

In the late course patients, though, what we see is much more shifting and blending, that is, a rapidly and constantly changing and infinitely variable [g] mix of

---

g "If we give no more examples, that is not because those already given represent adequately the multiplicity of the courses taken by manic-depressive insanity; it is absolutely inexhaustible."[169] Emil Kraepelin, 1921.

manic and depressive symptoms,[169] that is, a constantly shifting mixed episode.[189] So on one day (or week) a patient may have moderate depressive symptoms and mild manic symptoms, but on another day (or week) they may have minimal depressive symptoms and moderate to severe manic symptoms.

I would therefore support the adoption of the criteria for DMX developed by Akiskal, Benazzi, and others, that is, a major depressive episode, and at least 3 manic symptoms,[24,79] or preferably even the finding of Goldberg and others, that at least 2 manic symptoms indicate DMX.[13] I also support the adoption of the criteria for manic mixed episode (MMX, also described as "mixed mania") developed by McElroy and others, that is, a manic episode and at least 3 depressive symptoms.[71]

The patient and family can track these shifting mood and activation states (See Chapter 16) using a monthly mood chart (Figures 5.5 to 5.8), which takes only about 2 minutes per day to complete, and then the patient, the support person, and the clinician can get a clearer overview of the patient's constantly changing interplay of manic and depressive symptoms and occasional normal mood (called "euthymic") periods.

Figure 5.5

Date	1	2	3	4	5	6	7	8	9	10	11	12	13	14	15	16	17	18	19	20	21	22	23	24	25	26	27	28	29	30	31
Hours of Sleep																															

Over-Activation (Mania)

Severe
| Dysphoric Mania (Y/N) | | | | | | | | | | | | | | | | | | | | | | | | | | | | | | | |

High
| Essentially Incapacitated or Hospitalized | | | | | | | | | | | | | | | | | | | | | | | | | | | | | | | |

Moderate
| GREAT Difficulty with Goal-Oriented Ativity | | | | | | | | | | | | | | | | | | | | | | | | | | | | | | | |

Low
| SOME Difficulty with Goal-Oriented Activity | | | | | | | | | | | | | | | | | | | | | | | | | | | | | | | |

Mild
| More Energized & Productive with Little or No Functional Impairment | | | | | | | | | | | | | | | | | | | | | | | | | | | | | | | |

Normal Activation

Mild
| Normal / "Even" | | | | | | | | | | | | | | | | | | | | | | | | | | | | | | | |

Low
| Little or No Functional Impairment | | | | | | | | | | | | | | | | | | | | | | | | | | | | | | | |

Moderate
| Funtioning with SOME Effort | | | | | | | | | | | | | | | | | | | | | | | | | | | | | | | |

High
| Functioning with GREAT Effort | | | | | | | | | | | | | | | | | | | | | | | | | | | | | | | |

Severe
| Essentially Incapacitated or Hospitalized | | | | | | | | | | | | | | | | | | | | | | | | | | | | | | | |

Under-Activation and/or Sadness (Depression)

How to Record the Monthly Mood Chart Information in just Two Minutes a Day

1. Glance briefly over the blank Monthly Mood Chart, Figure 5.4, and make copies of Figure 5.4 as needed for your use. Next refer to the explanations as diagrammed in Figure 5.5.

2. Find the current day of the month in the list of numbers on the top edge of the blank form (Figure 5.4).

3. Figure out the total hours you actually slept last night (not just time in bed).

4. Enter this number just below yesterday's date.

5. At the end of the day today, think over whether you were mildly, moderately or highly over-activated (wound up, racy, edgy, energetic) today, and also whether you were mildly, moderately, or highly under-activated (draggy, slowed, sluggish, lacking in drive, energy, or motivation) and/or sad today.

6. Then enter either two check marks in the vertical column under today's date if you were both over-activated and under-activated/sad today, or only one check mark if you were only one of these, or if you felt even/"normal" today.

7. That's it! As you can see by comparing Figure 5.6 (December) with 5.7 (the following March), this very brief recording routine generates a lot of useful information over time. [h]

---

h In this particular example, the patient was on lithium treatment alone through December. At a visit after the December recording, we added divalproex/Depakote, with a very dramatic improvement in the patient's condition by the March recording.

Figure 5.6

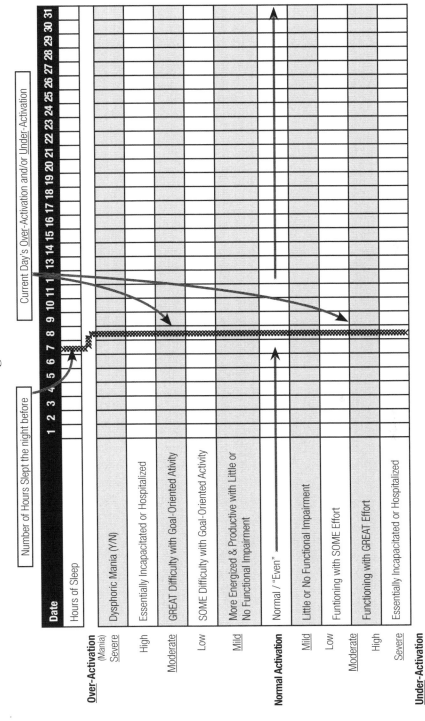

Figure 5.7

Date – DECEMBER 2011	1	2	3	4	5	6	7	8	9	10	11	12	13	14	15	16	17	18	19	20	21	22	23	24	25	26	27	28	29	30	31
Hours of Sleep	5	4	4	5	5	4	5	6	6	4	4	5	5	5	5	4	5	5	4	5	5	6	6	4	8	7	4	4	6	3	3

Over-Activation (Mania)

Severe — Dysphoric Mania (Y/N)																															
High — Essentially Incapacitated or Hospitalized			✓	✓	✓	✓																				✓					
Moderate — GREAT Difficulty with Goal-Oriented Ativity	✓						✓					✓												✓			✓			✓	
Low — SOME Difficulty with Goal-Oriented Activity																	✓	✓	✓	✓	✓										
Mild — More Energized & Productive with Little or No Functional Impairment								✓	✓																✓						✓

Normal Activation

Normal / "Even"					✓	✓							✓	✓	✓	✓	✓			✓	✓						✓	✓	✓		

Under-Activation and/or Sadness (Depression)

Mild — Little or No Functional Impairment										✓	✓	✓											✓								
Low — Funtioning with SOME Effort										✓														✓							
Moderate — Functioning with GREAT Effort																															
Severe — Essentially Incapacitated or Hospitalized																															

Figure 5.8

Date – MARCH 2012	1	2	3	4	5	6	7	8	9	10	11	12	13	14	15	16	17	18	19	20	21	22	23	24	25	26	27	28	29	30	31
Hours of Sleep	6	6	5	5	5	5	6	6	6	6	6	6	6	6	6	4	4	6	6	5	5	5	5	5	5	5	5	4	4	4	5

Over-Activation (Mania)

	1	2	3	4	5	6	7	8	9	10	11	12	13	14	15	16	17	18	19	20	21	22	23	24	25	26	27	28	29	30	31
Severe — Dysphoric Mania (Y/N)																															
High — Essentially Incapacitated or Hospitalized		✓	✓																												
Moderate — GREAT Difficulty with Goal-Oriented Ativity																															
Low — SOME Difficulty with Goal-Oriented Activity														✓	✓																
Mild — More Energized & Productive with Little or No Functional Impairment						✓							✓									✓	✓	✓		✓	✓	✓	✓		✓

Normal Activation

	1	2	3	4	5	6	7	8	9	10	11	12	13	14	15	16	17	18	19	20	21	22	23	24	25	26	27	28	29	30	31
Normal / "Even"				✓	✓	✓	✓	✓	✓	✓	✓	✓	✓					✓	✓	✓	✓				✓					✓	
Mild — Little or No Functional Impairment			✓	✓	✓																										
Low — Funtioning with SOME Effort																															
Moderate — Functioning with GREAT Effort																															
High — Functioning with GREAT Effort																															
Severe — Essentially Incapacitated or Hospitalized																															

Under-Activation and/or Sadness (Depression)

51

The DSM-IV-TR[24] description of mixed episode as involving a picture-perfect 50-50 split of manic and depressive symptoms, both of moderate-to-severe intensity consistently for a full week, is something more likely seen in diagnostic manuals than in actual patients, and thus has possible theoretical value, but very little clinical value.

By the time the patient is in the late course, the depressive mixed episode (DMX) has moved in and taken over as the most frequent presentation of bipolar disorder, almost three times more common in my experience than pure bipolar depression, as depicted in Figure 5.9 below:

Figure 5.9

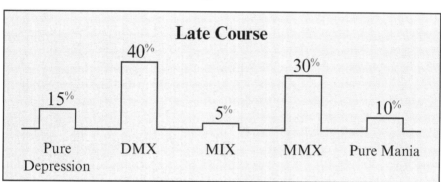

As noted, almost every bipolar patient visit to the psychiatrist begins with the patient complaining of what they honestly perceive and report to be depression. This sometimes however involves primarily situational or economic or relationship worries or troubles that don't even meet criteria for a full major depressive episode.[11,24] (A major depressive episode is a full 2 weeks of very disruptive down mood interfering with functioning in several areas.[24] See Appendix.)

Of bipolar patients who actually meet criteria for a major depressive episode, careful evaluation[69,94] shows that most of these patients are actually presenting instead with a depressive mixed episode/DMX,[79,80] a clinically useful predictor that they are not likely to respond well to the addition of a regular antidepressant as a means of treating their depressive mixed state.[13,68]

Contrast the above percentages with how we might have divided the same pie if we had instead applied the DSM-IV-TR[24] criteria, which sharply limit mixed episode (and thereby enormously exaggerate the percentage of "bipolar depression"):

Figure 5.10

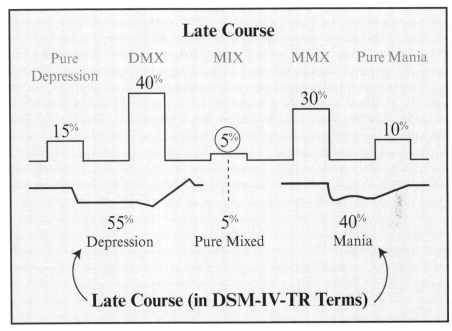

Looking at it this way, clinicians might be tempted to treat over half (55%) of late course bipolar I and II patients with antidepressants and continue them on these as maintenance treatment. (Interestingly, this is similar to the percentage of U.S. bipolar I and II patients treated with antidepressants long-term [50% to 84%].[8,9,64])

This creates problems, however, because the vast majority of good quality clinical research shows that only a very small minority of bipolar depressed patients, about 1 in 6 (or about 15% to 16%) are likely to benefit from treatment with ADs for longer than 3 months.[15,16,19,20,21,30,42,82] This DSM-IV-TR polarity-based view of the bipolar I and II episode spectrum, that is, broadly-defined depressive episodes and extremely narrowly defined mixed episodes, may perhaps in part explain why we American clinicians (more so than our European counterparts[12,21]) prescribe ADs as a maintenance treatment to roughly two-thirds of bipolar I and II patients,[8,9,64] "with extremely low success rates."[21]

Operating with the same very narrow DSM-IV-TR[24] definition of mixed episode and the same broad definition of bipolar depressive episode, the recently-published largest meta-analysis of the effectiveness of short-term antidepressant treatment (less than 4 months) for acute bipolar depression showed that "antidepressants were not statistically superior to placebo or other current standard treatment for bipolar depression."[29] That is, there was *no* benefit whatsoever from AD medicine, whether combined with MSs or not, even in the short-term treatment of bipolar depression. This goes somewhat against the expectation that we would get *at least something* from the antidepressants, at least acutely. It is, however, consistent with a prospective recent study looking at a similar question,[18] that also showed *no* benefit whatsoever during up to 6 months of adding antidepressants to mood stabilizer treatment for bipolar depressed patients (as compared to adding placebo to the mood stabilizer).

Interestingly, it may be precisely because of the way the DSM-IV-TR slices the bipolar disorder pie that these studies failed to show any benefit whatsoever from the addition of antidepressants. If instead, 'patients with bipolar depression' had been selected with the broader view of mixed episode that I and many others have suggested,[69,73,79,80,82,94,118,171] we might have been treating 15% of the overall bipolar sample (i.e., those with pure bipolar depression) rather than 55%, as suggested by DSM-IV-TR.[24] We might have limited the subjects to those with pure bipolar depression, i.e., depression with less than 2 manic symptoms.[13] We would have excluded those with depressive mixed episode (DMX, about 40% of the overall bipolar sample), who in clinical practice get worse rather than better with the addition of antidepressants,[13,68] if they show any change at all.

Given the above, one can readily see that the broader definition of mixed episode (with a narrower definition of pure bipolar depressive episode) provides a wealth of clinical information missing from the pure DSM-IV-TR[24] categories, which instead offer an over-broad description of bipolar depressive episode.[57,69]

That is, if one uses the DSM-IV-TR approach to diagnosing bipolar depression for selection of patients for whom to add unipolar ADs to their mood stabilizers as maintenance treatment, one is likely to include a huge swath of patients with depressive mixed episode (DMX), and end up doing more harm than good, as in so many of the above studies.

Researchers have been looking for decades for the possibility of ADs triggering manic or hypomanic episodes during research studies, but manic or hypomanic "switches" due to ADs are often not seen in short-term clinical trials. This is, on the surface, somewhat surprising. By way of comparison, 44% of patients in the STEP-BD study self-reported having had the prior experience of switches into mania or hypomania linked to past AD use, and very interestingly the switches in this study were correlated with multiple past antidepressant trials.[37]

In contrast to recent studies not seeing increases in new mania with the addition of antidepressants, are the somewhat surprising recent findings that bipolar patients who were on antidepressants had more frequent and more severe depressive episodes[12,25,26] than bipolar patients who were not on antidepressants. Bipolar patients with only 2 or 3 manic symptoms (that is, with depressive mixed episode, DMX) had worse manic symptoms even by 3 months with the addition of antidepressants,[13,68] i.e., worsening of their depressive mixed episodes. If antidepressants are associated with worsening of mixed episodes, this may account for the finding of more suicidal behaviors in bipolar patients being treated with antidepressants,[38] as mixed episodes are known to be associated with more suicidal thoughts and behaviors.[59,94,110,118,170]

Bipolar patients who had rapid cycling have also been noted to experience worsening of rapid cycling after antidepressants were added.[27] In another recent study, patients with rapid cycling who were continued on antidepressants had worse rapid cycling that those whose antidepressants were tapered and discontinued.[19] Patients with many courses of antidepressant medication treatment were also found to have more suicidal thoughts and actions,[59] and less ability to respond well to later treatment efforts.[60]

With the awareness of the natural history of the disorder, however, these "surprises" would all make perfect sense. It takes 5 to 16 years from the beginning of bipolar illness to eventual correct diagnosis. During this time, most patients are diagnosed as having major depressive disorder instead.[58,63-66] As a result, they are often subjected to multiple antidepressant trials during this interval, and the 5 to 16 year interval is generally long enough for the patient's illness to progress from the early course to the late course.[57,58] (Patient characteristics shown in large research studies show that patients have generally already had 10 to 20 years of illness before entering the studies.[211]) This then increases the odds that by the time they are identified and entered into research studies, they are already in the late course of bipolar disorder.

Therefore, any worsening seen when adding ADs during the research studies might not manifest as simple manic or hypomanic episodes, which are instead seen much more often in the early course of the disorder, as described in the previous chapter.

Instead, worsening associated with the new addition of antidepressants might be expected to manifest in such studies as worse late course symptoms and episodes, i.e., worse mixed episodes, worse rapid cycling, and worse depression.

Therefore, in my opinion, two of the keys to greater success in the treatment of bipolar disorder are first, the renewed recognition of cycling and recurrence as its central features[4] (rather than polarity), and second, the recognition of the greater clinical usefulness of the broader view of mixed states[4]. Without the first of these, we can't understand bipolar disorder at all. Without the second, we fail to understand the extremely common and very important late course of the illness.[21]

Section B:

Key Medication Treatment Issues

Chapter 6

Duffy's Rule

Restoring sleep and the sleep-wake cycle is perhaps the most important task of bipolar disorder treatment.

This chapter begins with Duffy's (and others') Rule, which describes how sleep and the sleep-wake cycle are relatively dominant forces in the course and successful treatment of bipolar disorder.[56,137,194]

Duffy's Rule: In a well established bipolar patient, the number of hours of sleep per 24 hours is the single most reliable indicator of the current mood state, that is, manic or mixed vs. depressed.

For instance, patients with pure bipolar depressions are very sluggish and draggy. They often move slowly, think slowly, and speak slowly.[131,154,182] They tend to sleep remarkably long hours.[131,138,154,182,199] A patient with pure bipolar depression can easily sleep 10 to 20 hours per 24 hours, and can often accomplish almost nothing whatsoever during the day, sometimes for days or weeks on end. Therefore if you have a patient with a very convincing diagnosis of bipolar I or II disorder, and they're sleeping 11 or more hours per 24 for days on end, the diagnosis is likely pure bipolar depression.

If, on the other hand, you have a bipolar patient sleeping 5 or less hours per night for several days, pure bipolar depression is pretty much out of the question, and you're much more likely working with a patient in a manic or mixed state.[i]

---

i Please note that insomnia alone is not enough to make the diagnosis of bipolar mania in the first place. One needs additional symptoms as listed in the DSM-V-TR,[24] see Appendix.

The rule seems too simple, but it works almost every time. It seems less obvious to many clinicians because they hear "depression" early in the interview, and are writing the prescription for "antidepressants" before they've spent the time asking and discovering the manic symptoms in detail, especially the number of hours of sleep per 24 hours. The history taking needs to include hearing the story from the patient's closest support person, who is probably having a lot more trouble with the patient's manic symptoms than the patient is.

But once you learn Duffy's Rule, you won't be fooled nearly as easily ever again. It's not that the patients are consciously trying to fool the clinicians, but bipolar patients just don't usually view the manic symptoms as much of a problem at all, in contrast to the depressive symptoms, which they hate. Many times it's someone else who's picking up the pieces after the manic or mixed episode rather than the patient himself (or herself).

To summarize:

1. If a reliably-diagnosed bipolar I or II patient is sleeping 5 hours per night or less for days at a time, the diagnosis is most likely manic or mixed episode.

2. If a similar patient is sleeping 11 or more hours per 24 hours for days on end, the diagnosis is most likely pure bipolar depressive episode.

After missing bipolar disorder altogether, misdiagnosing depressive mixed episodes as bipolar depression and treating with ADs, is one of the most common wild goose chases we clinicians go on. Treating mixed episodes with ADs hardly ever leads to lasting overall improvement, but it seems to have a fairly good chance of making the mixed episode worse.

The ones who suffer, though, are usually not the clinicians, but the patients and their families. We can easily avoid this detour if we remember Duffy's Rule and remember to determine, with outside observation and confirmation, how many hours per 24 our bipolar patients are actually sleeping.

On the therapeutic side, the first order of business is restoring patients to a full 6 to 10 hours per night of uninterrupted good quality sleep.[194] If one can aggressively pursue and achieve this, all sorts of other good things start to fall into place very rapidly. If, on the other hand, one fails to achieve significant improvement in sleep and the sleep-wake cycle, the patient has little chance of getting well, so what else could possibly be more important?

Bipolar disorder is, in a very real sense, a disorder of daily rhythms ("circadian rhythms"), such as the sleep-wake cycle.[194] For this reason, unless the patient is working on the night shift, it is quite important that the patient gets a full night's sleep at night, and be active, productive, and socially connected during the day, as part of developing "lifestyle regularity" and regular daily biological rhythms.[86,144,171]

Therefore any of the sedative medications we give, such as mood stabilizers or antipsychotics (or any tranquilizers that are still in the medication list and haven't yet been phased out) should be given primarily at or near bedtime. Alternative options include 1/3 at supper and 2/3 at bedtime, or 1/3 during the day and 2/3 at night.

Fellow clinicians sometimes ask, "But what about maintaining adequate therapeutic blood levels throughout the whole 24 hours?" Hospital regimens tend to dose such medicines "b.i.d.," i.e., "twice a day," with half the total dose in the morning and half at night, presumably for just this reason.

This is an extremely widespread practice, and in certain systemic or blood-borne infections, maintaining smooth, high blood levels of the antibiotic(s) is very important, so as to have adequate/"minimum inhibitory" concentrations of the antibiotic to clear the infection.

However, if one tries to translate this reasoning to bipolar disorder, it causes problems. Patients treated with such regimens, with 1/2 the dose of sedative medication in the morning, doze off halfway through the morning with a long nap and therefore don't sleep nearly as well at night. If the clinician doesn't get the patient sleeping continuously through the night, and then up and alert throughout the day, all the even, therapeutic blood levels in the world aren't going to do a bit of good, and the patient simply won't get well. And, if the clinician sedates the patient heavily during the day, they'll hate it, and they'll stop the medicine the first chance they get.

Case 6.1

Ms. B, a career woman in her mid 40s with known and previously treated bipolar disorder, consulted a psychiatrist who treated her for the next 10 years with lithium carbonate extended release 450 mg twice a day morning and night, Zoloft/sertraline 100 mg every morning, and trazodone 100 mg every night. Over this ten years she continued to experience serious mood cycling which caused major problems with her professional career and her relationships.

Ms. B also experienced disruptive daytime drowsiness from the morning lithium dose, and she therefore asked the psychiatrist if it was really necessary to take the lithium on a twice a day schedule, which he told her it was.

The patient, then in her mid 50s, sought out a different psychiatrist, who noted on the initial evaluation that she was mildly to moderately manic, with the manic symptoms still increasing. Ms. B also told the new psychiatrist that past manias had caused significant damage to career and relationships. As part of the currently accelerating mania, the patient reported racing thoughts, distractibility, edginess, irritability, impulsivity, and only being able to get 6 hours of broken sleep per night.

Accordingly, the new psychiatrist switched her lithium all to the night dose, in an attempt both to improve sleep and reduce the daytime sedation. He ordered a lithium level, and based on the result, he reduced her total lithium dose to 675 mg/day, all given at night .

Given that Ms. B arrived with an accelerating manic episode, the new psychiatrist also discussed with her the need to start tapering her antidepressant (AD, Zoloft), and together they started a very gradual taper as described in Chapter 10.

When seen for a follow-up appointment 6 months later, Ms. B was taking all her lithium at night, and her AD dose (of Zoloft) had been gradually reduced to 50% of the original dose. Ms. B's sleep had now improved to 6 to 8 hours of good-quality, uninterrupted sleep per night. She was waking up rested, and her daytime energy had returned to normal. She came to this appointment calm, beaming, and completely free of any recent manic or depressive symptoms.

Therefore my advice to the clinician is to load sedative effects toward a full night of sleep. If you restore the normal sleep-wake cycle, with full activity during the day, the patient is much more likely to recover.

Chapter 7

C A L M   S E A S:

An easy way to remember
the main bipolar treatment issues

This chapter starts with the letters and core treatment issues from a memory device (to help remember key bipolar disorder treatment issues) first described in a 2008 letter to the editor I co-authored with S. Nassir Ghaemi, M.D., M.P.H. (CALM[33]), and which we then expanded in 2011 (CALM SEA[43]). I recently added the final S to remind us of the serious risks of stimulants and stress. The current chapter then goes on to describe these treatment issues in the web of the broader topics discussed throughout the book.

C: Control the manic and mixed symptoms first as a way to start to control the cycling.[33,43,152]

Patients often suffer with insomnia, irritability, edginess, high anxiety, racing thoughts, impulsivity, inability to concentrate, inability to function, and/or high-risk behaviors. These high-risk behaviors are generally out of character for the patient, and may include excessive spending, driving recklessly and too fast, alcohol and drug abuse, and excessive and ill-advised sexual behavior. These untreated or undertreated manic symptoms often lead to tension in the patients' relationships and fairly often, to outright loss of their relationships. They also lead to job tensions, and fairly commonly to job loss, major financial pressures, legal problems, etc.

That is, due to the untreated or undertreated manic symptoms, the patients are burning their bridges and making their overall life situations that much more difficult. This is part of the reason it is so crucial to look more actively for manic symptoms from the very beginning, and to treat them rapidly and successfully.

As you'll see on reading the rest of the book, if you don't discover and control the manic and mixed symptoms early on, you won't be able to calm the cycling. And if you don't calm the cycling, you have no chance whatsoever to reduce the depressive symptoms over the long term anyway.

A: **A**ntidepressant medicines: Use sparingly, and only as part of evidence-based (scientifically proven) strategies.[6]

The conventional antidepressant medications (unipolar antidepressants) are pretty good at treating major depressive disorder[11,24] ("regular depression" or "unipolar" depression, with no history of manias ever), but they don't work very often in bipolar disorder.

L: **L**ong-term view:

This is a lifelong disorder, which changes significantly over the natural life history of the disorder. In order to treat the disorder successfully, one must be very familiar with its natural history, which is described in Chapters 4 and 5.

M: **M**ood stabilizers:

The most important medicines in the treatment of bipolar disorder are the "Big Three" traditional mood stabilizers lithium (Eskalith, LithoBID, and others), divalproex (Depakote and others), and carbamazepine (Equetro, Tegretol, and others).[20,41] The overall next most useful medicine is the newer traditional mood stabilizer lamotrigine (Lamictal), which has a very different range of effectiveness.[61] You will see that these medicines are heavily emphasized in Chapter 8, on where the individual mood stabilizers work, and in Chapter 9, on building effective bipolar disorder medicine regimens.

S: Sleep:

Restoring normal sleep and the normal sleep-wake cycle is one of the biggest keys to success. Consistent full-duration (6 to 10 hours per night), uninterrupted, refreshing sleep at the right time in the 24-hour cycle is one of the key elements of successful recovery in bipolar disorder. In contrast, sleep deprivation is both a cause of new bipolar mood episodes, as well as a result of, and a marker for, mania.[137]

E: Endocrine/Metabolic

Endocrine and metabolic factors are very important, and are easily remembered as "TSH" (which just happens to be the same letters as the single most useful thyroid screening test, Thyroid Stimulating Hormone):

T   Thyroid state plays a major role in bipolar disorder and in its successful treatment.[5,20,49,139,149]

S   Too much or too little Steroid (from internal or external sources, including anabolic steroids used by body builders or prescribed steroids for medical conditions[90]) may trigger bipolar mood episodes, most commonly manic or mixed episodes, and sometimes with psychosis, confusion, depression, panic, and/or suicidal behaviors.[90]

H   Hormonal shifts, such as onset of menstrual periods, puberty, pregnancy, delivery, menopause, and even monthly premenstrual changes[142] may be associated with the start of bipolar mood episodes, or with greater frequency of bipolar mood episodes.

A: Activity:

Consistently getting a full day's vigorous physical, mental, and social Activity at the right time of day helps stabilize the crucial sleep-wake cycle, and also adds meaning and purpose to one's life.

S: 2 more **S**s:

Stress (including life crises or medical events, see case example below), and Stimulants (including cocaine, crack, methamphetamine, diet pills, high-dose ADHD medications, or even high-dose caffeine) may also trigger bipolar mood episodes, most commonly manic or mixed episodes, sometimes with psychosis.

Case 7.1: A woman in her late 80s, with no prior history of bipolar disorder, was clear-headed, medically relatively well, and able to live semi-independently. She then suffered a heart attack.

Over the next 6 to 8 weeks she developed a full manic episode, with pronounced insomnia, talking too much and too fast, thoughts racing and all jumbled up, writing excessively, and finally so disorganized she could suddenly no longer manage her affairs and had to be hospitalized. She had emergency psychiatric consultation and follow-up, and was treated with divalproex (Depakote) and olanzapine (Zyprexa), with gradual clearing of her mania over the course of the following month.

Chapter 8

Ceilings, Cores, and Floors:

Where and how do the individual mood stabilizers work?

This chapter describes how the individual **traditional mood stabilizers** (MSs: lithium, divalproex [Depakote and others], carbamazepine [Equetro, Tegretol, and others], and lamotrigine [Lamictal]) work.

We'll discuss which ones work better as **ceilings** to contain manic and mixed episodes and symptoms "from above."[36] This includes lithium, divalproex, carbamazepine, and to a lesser extent, lamotrigine. That is, lamotrigine exerts only weak anti-manic effects,[61,123,124] whereas the other three mood stabilizers exert strong anti-manic effects. See Table 8.1 below, which summarizes the actions of the traditional mood stabilizers.

Table 8.1

Mood Stabilizer Efficacy				
	Lithium	Divalproex	Carbamazepine	Lamotrigine
"Ceiling" (vs. Manic/Mixed)	Strong	Strong	Strong	Weak
"Core" (Maintenance)	Strong	Moderate to Strong	Moderate?	Moderate to Strong
"Floor" (Acute Depression)	Weak to Moderate	Weak?	Weak?	Weak to Moderate
"Floor" (Maintenance vs. Depression)	Weak to Moderate	Weak?	Weak?	Strong
Suicide Prevention	Strong	Some? (1 study [141])	None	None

Roger Sparhawk, M.D., 2012.

If patients do not tolerate lithium, divalproex, or carbamazepine, we may instead try oxcarbazepine/Trileptal (so long as the patient doesn't have an allergy to its chemical cousin carbamazepine). The evidence for the use of oxcarbazepine, however, is relatively weak.

Otherwise we might use the newer, "atypical antipsychotics" (AAPs) as anti-manic **ceilings**, with or without traditional MSs, especially if we need very rapid anti-manic effects. All but the very newest of the AAPs (see Glossary) have been shown to be effective against manic and mixed episodes. For most patients with bipolar I or II disorder, however, they are likely to be more effective when they are prescribed without ADs:

Case 8.1

A woman in her 50s had suffered with and been treated for bipolar disorder for 14 years, the first 4 years with simpler early course episodes (see Chapter 4), and the last 10 years with more complex late course mixed episodes and more rapid cycling, as described in Chapters 4 and 5.

Over the first 12 years of her treatment she had been cared for by a number of clinicians, for a couple of years by primary doctors, and then by psychiatrists.

She had been treated for most of that time with atypical antipsychotics. During all of that 12 years, however, she was treated continuously with various antidepressants (ADs), even during and after hospitalizations for manic and mixed episodes. During that 12 years she never experienced complete clearing of major mood episodes.

Then for the most recent 2 years of her treatment, she saw a nurse practitioner, who took her off the ADs. The nurse practitioner remodeled the patient's regimen eventually to 2 atypical antipsychotics and the newer mood stabilizer lamotrigine ("floor"), and no ADs. Over the last year or so on this regimen, the patient remained stable without any major mood episodes for the first time since her treatment started 14 years earlier.

Interestingly, the patient was never tried during the course of her 14 years of treatment on lithium, divalproex, or carbamazepine, which are 3 of the 4 medicines with the highest likelihood of successful treatment.[20]

We'll also need to understand which MSs provide "stabilization from below."[36] Lamotrigine and lithium have demonstrated effectiveness as floors. The AAPs quetiapine (Seroquel XR) and olanzapine (Zyprexa), the olanzapine-fluoxetine combination (OFC, Symbyax), thyroid augmentation with T3 or T4, and just recently, lurasidone (Latuda),[213,215,216] have also demonstrated benefit as "floors." Their role in treating bipolar depression and depressive mixed episodes (DMX) is discussed in the next chapter. Ziprasidone (Geodon) was just recently the very first treatment tested specifically for depressive mixed episode (DMX), and this randomized clinical trial showed ziprasidone to be extremely effective for DMX.[218] **Floors** reduce the downward/depressive swings of the mood cycling. Lamotrigine is more effective in preventing future downward swings than in acutely treating current depressive episodes. It has, however, shown some effectiveness against acute/current depressive episodes if these are severe.[124]

This chapter began at the 2011 International Conference on Bipolar Disorders in Pittsburgh,[91] where I met a couple of psychiatric residents (see Glossary) who were very much interested in what they had just been learning of the considerable effectiveness of the traditional mood stabilizers.

As at most residency programs across the country,[92] they had been taught very little about the MSs up to that point. Perhaps an even bigger problem is that in the majority of residency programs throughout the United States,[92] psychiatric residents don't get to see faculty members model and explain using traditional MSs with confidence in a majority of their bipolar patients, and with the solid conviction that the MSs will do a lot of the heavy lifting in treating bipolar disorder. This is very possibly because most of the faculty don't have this confidence and conviction.[8,9,92]

At any rate, after thinking over the new information they were hearing at the conference, these residents were eager to learn more, and asked, "Is there a way to help residents become more comfortable with starting mood stabilizers, rather than rely on antipsychotics for mania?"[93]

I strongly suspect that many patients and families would be curious about this topic as well, and therefore this chapter attempts to tell about mood cycling and the use of MSs in a series of easy-to-understand descriptions and a few pictures explaining treatment from above and below,[36] and even seemingly from within the cycling.

To show mood cycling in a visual way, we're going to apply the image from the memory device CALM SEAS by imagining mood states as if they were the surface of a pond (or sea), and we'd like to keep the surface of the pond relatively smooth and calm. We'll start with a chart showing someone who does not have bipolar disorder, this would be a relatively smooth line near the "normal" center line, but with some fairly mild movements up and down over time, as almost all of us experience some mild up and down times over the course of our lives.

Figure 8.1

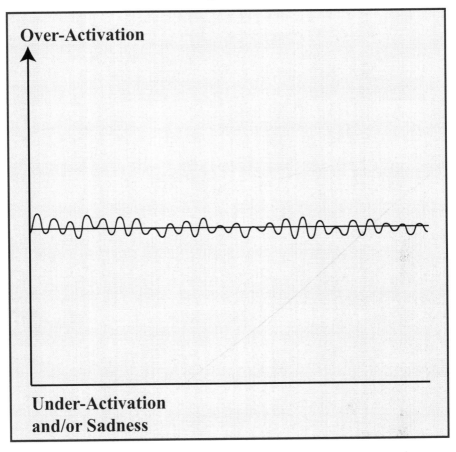

If we wanted to picture the mood states of someone with bipolar disorder, we could show higher states of mood, energy, and "activation" (where the patient is wound up, and not sleeping much) as being waves above the horizontal center line. Lower states of mood, energy, and activation (and usually excessive sleep) are shown as waves below the line. The more extreme the mood states, the farther the waves will be from the horizontal center line.

We'll then start with the first diagram and add a line with some fairly big waves to represent the mood, energy, and activation states of someone with bipolar disorder.

Figure 8.2

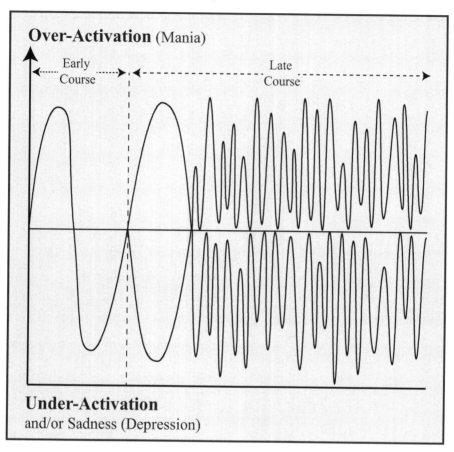

In the above diagram, the early course (see Chapter 4) consists of more simple manias and depressions. The late course (see Chapters 4 and 5) consists of mixed episodes and rapid cycling. The late course is depicted above (moving left to right over time) first as a simple mixed episode, then as rapid, ultra-rapid, or ultradian cycling [j] in the form of a rapidly shifting mixed episode (see also Figure 4.4), which is what a high percentage of late course patients have when

---

[j] Mixed episodes appear, along with the development of rapid cycling (four or more illness episodes per year, as represented schematically also in Figure 4.1), to be the standard features of the bipolar disorder late course.[21] Many patients in the late course experience cycling much more rapid than rapid cycling, such as "ultra-rapid cycling," that is multiple distinct mood episodes within a week[5] (as shown also in Figure 4.2), or even "ultradian cycling," which is multiple mood episodes within the same day[4,6] (Figure 4.3).

they come to my office for the first time.

Compared to moderate highs and lows, the more extreme mood, energy, and activation states are generally more damaging to the patient's lives and relationships, and these are now noted on the following diagram.

Figure 8.3

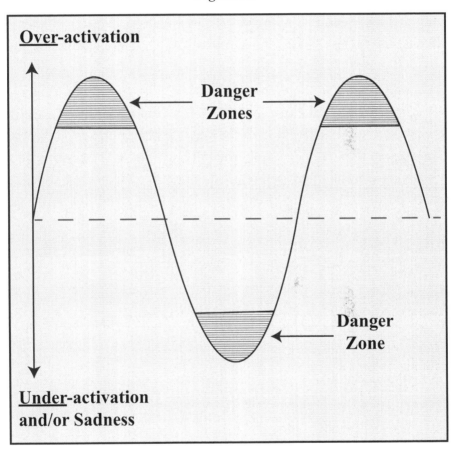

At the extreme highs, patients often have insomnia, racing thoughts, poor concentration, poor judgment, irritability, talking too much and too loudly, more arguments, anxiety, unrealistic, impulsive and poorly considered decisions and actions, and high-risk behaviors. The high-risk behaviors may include driving way too fast, getting into physical fights, spending way too much money (sometimes for things they don't even need), doing street drugs and/or drinking way too much, becoming more sexual than usual or even promiscuous, and getting arrested and thrown into jail or psychiatric hospital for out of control behaviors. These high-risk behaviors are very much different from how these same patients would normally operate when they were well.

Sometimes while "up," patients may decide that they are doing terrific, or feel better than they've ever felt. They may then decide that they're obviously "cured" and don't need their medicines; so they stop their medicines without first discussing it with their doctors, whom they now feel they no longer need.

The above behaviors often wear out their spouses, partners, family, and friends, and lead to relationship break-ups and loss of social supports, which may make the patient's eventual recovery that much more difficult. The above behaviors also often lead to patients being fired from their jobs, or impulsively walking off and losing their jobs. They may also miss doctors' appointments, and not comply with treatment, leading in some cases to the doctors dismissing them from treatment.

In summary, the patients lose control of their mood, thinking, judgment, and behavior, and run the serious risk of burning most or all of their bridges, so that the eventual recovery and rebuilding of their lives becomes that much more difficult. You can see that it is crucial to bring this stuff under control as quickly as possible, before the patients destroy much of their lives.

At the extreme lows, by contrast, patients are as if spray-painted on the couch or bed. They are extremely under-activated, if you will. They sleep 12 to 20 hours per 24 hours, and much of the rest of the time is spent on the couch, bed, or floor, just lying there and hoping the bad feeling will go away. They have no interest or energy for anything. They don't enjoy anything, and they don't seem to be able to do anything. They don't usually get into fights, but they may get fired from work for calling in sick too often or just not showing up.

If this goes on too long, those around them may give up on them. As you may have already seen in Chapter 5, this state, pure bipolar depression, is present in only about 15% to 20% of patients coming to the psychiatrist, and its treatment is a special situation described in Chapter 9. Suicide risk is often discussed with regard to bipolar depression, but may be even greater with mixed episodes.[110,147]

Some of the other bipolar patients reporting feelings of depression are actually just very drowsy and tired from the sedative effects of the medicines or (sometimes pretty large) medicine combinations they're taking, as described in Chapters 3, 6, and 15.

Many others are instead actually suffering with so-called "mixed" episodes, with a mix of high and low states of mood, energy, and activation, as shown in Figure 8.4 (and also discussed in Chapters 4 and 5).

Figure 8.4

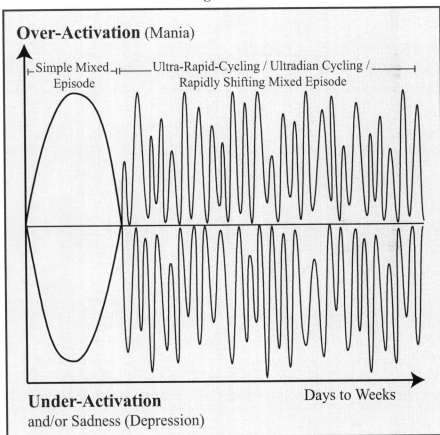

"Depression" is almost always the patient's presenting complaint.[44,69,72,94] On the other hand, if you learn how to ask symptoms carefully and in detail and to get collateral history from close observers, mixed episode is by far the most common presenting mood state.[44,69,72,94,147]

It would be really nice if we had magical devices something like magnets that worked from the horizontal center line ("Normal"), and exerted their pull on the surface of the water itself, pulling the surface back down toward normal when it started to go too high, and pulling the surface back up toward normal when it started to go too low. Fortunately, we do have "magnets" like that in the real world, and they're called mood stabilizers (MSs). When we treat patients with MSs in studies compared with patients treated with placebo (an inactive sugar pill), the patients on the MSs go for longer periods of time without going too high or too low, that is, into a high or low mood episode, as compared with the patients who were randomly assigned to the placebo group.[103,104] I call this property **core** stabilization, as it seems to keep moods and activation in the center zone, and also spread out the mood/activation episodes over time, so that they occur more slowly and less frequently, as shown in Figure 8.5 below.

Figure 8.5

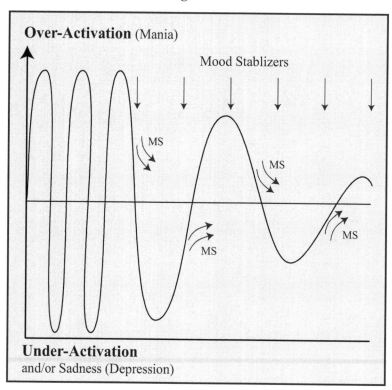

Core stabilization differs from the ceilings and floors we use, which seem to push down from above, or up from below. All four of the mood stabilizers provide core stabilization, some perhaps more than others, as described below (and in Table 8.1 above).

Lithium is the best-established core mood stabilizer (and also has some antidepressant activity). Divalproex has the second-best level of evidence, and carbamazepine has perhaps the weakest documentation as a core mood stabilizer. All three of them are effective for controlling over-activation; that is, they function as **ceilings**, or anti-manics.[104] Lamotrigine is a more recently discovered core mood stabilizer, and is unique in providing more of an antidepressant maintenance **floor** than the others, but not very much anti-manic ceiling.[103]

We will go on to describe how these agents can be used to build effective bipolar disorder treatment medicine combinations (regimens) in the next chapter.

Chapter 9

Building Effective Bipolar Regimens (Medication Combinations), From the General to the Specific

Descriptions of how to build regimens are generally derived from guidelines agreed upon by expert consensus panels.[95,96,108,213] Many such guidelines are now a few years old. They tend to stay as close as possible to the evidence from clinical trials and other studies in the scientific literature. Since there is much more available evidence about short-term treatment,[k] the guidelines tend to focus more on how to treat the various mood states over the short term. In trying to stay close to the evidence, they also tend to focus more on the specific mood states than on a general approach to treating bipolar disorder.

In this chapter we're going to take just the opposite approach, that is, moving from the general to the specific. We will also start with the long-term treatment issues, before moving to the acute treatment of specific mood states. This is done so that patients, families, and clinicians can start the immediate treatment with the long-term strategy clearly in mind.[143,190] This follows Stephen Covey's idea, as written in *The Seven Habits of Highly Effective People,* "Begin with

---

k This may be because clinical research is very expensive, and longer-term trials are then even more expensive. This may also explain why there are many more FDA approvals for short-term acute treatment than for long-term maintenance.

the end in mind."[97] If we don't keep a clear idea of the long-term aim, we finds ourselves being bounced around from one crisis and one mood state and one acute treatment to the other without any long-term vision, that is, with no rudder to guide the ship of treatment.

We now proceed to the treatment model.

A. A Sequential Model for Building Successful Long-Term Bipolar Disorder Treatment Regimens:

We will begin building our hypothetical general long-term bipolar regimen as follows, by starting with the very best proven medicines first:

1. One of the traditional core mood stabilizers, i.e., lithium, divalproex, carbamazepine, or lamotrigine, in the absence of "antidepressant" medications.

Note that in "Treatment As Usual in the community" (TAU, to be discussed below), the above mood stabilizers are either not started, or are started after antidepressant (AD) medications, and often after multiple trials of AD medications, without ever discontinuing the AD medications when the mood stabilizers are added. This leads in such cases to invalid trials of the mood stabilizers (MSs), as the MSs are often much more effective when prescribed without AD medications.

Choice # 2 is thus listed as follows:

2. NO "ANTIDEPRESSANT" MEDICATION (i.e., no conventional/ unipolar antidepressants).

Entry #2 may seem an unnecessary repetition of #1, but unfortunately most U.S. prescribers and/or patients and families either aren't aware of what was stated in #1, assume that "in the absence of antidepressant medication" must be a typo, or don't believe it, despite what is now fairly overwhelming evidence in support of leaving out the antidepressant medicines.

Of course, as noted previously, any change in your own treatment needs to be worked out with, and directed by your own treating clinician.

I often ask my bipolar patients which medicines they've taken over the years and record these. Usually they give me a long and unbroken string of three to twelve ADs stretching back five to twenty-five years, often combined with antipsychotics, primarily the AAPs.

Here and there they may have been tried on a traditional mood stabilizer, but often these mood stabilizer trials are abandoned as treatment failures, with neither patient nor clinician being aware that continuing the antidepressant during the mood stabilizer trial renders the trial meaningless.

I then often ask the patient if they've been on "the best AD" yet, and they're usually bewildered and ask, "Which one is that?" They seem to be fully expecting me to name yet another AD. They're just as bewildered at my reply: "No antidepressant." Remember however that getting to "No AD" is a tricky business, and some considerations for this potentially risky passage are discussed in Chapter 10.

We now move on to sequential additions **#3, 4, and 5,** to the generic template of bipolar disorder treatment options:

3. Add[103,104] or switch to a second traditional MS (lithium, divalproex, carbamazepine, or lamotrigine, depending on mood state) or an AAP (atypical antipsychotic), thyroid augmentation, or psychotherapy (including possibly a psychotherapy specifically shown to establish lifestyle regularity[86,144,153] and to benefit the recovery of bipolar patients, such as IPSRT [InterPersonal and Social Rhythms Therapy][86,144,153]).

4. Add (or switch to a different) AAP or a second or third MS, thyroid augmentation, psychotherapy, omega-3/fish oil,[151] or adjunctive medication (e.g. zolpidem or eszopiclone or temazepam or other sedative-hypnotic for insomnia, or benzodiazepine or gabapentin for anxiety and/or insomnia).

5. Add (or switch to a different) AAP, third or fourth MS, Seroquel XR (quetiapine), olanzapine (Zyprexa), olanzapine-fluoxetine combination (OFC), thyroid augmentation, lurasidone (Latuda),[215,216] psychotherapy, pramipexole,[195,196] modafinil, omega-3/fish oil, unipolar antidepressant,

haloperidol or other older antipsychotic, or adjunctive medication (as in #4 above), or hospitalization with or without ECT (electro-convulsive treatment).

Here we have now the full sequential model in one place:

1. Lithium, divalproex, carbamazepine, or lamotrigine in the absence of "antidepressant" medication.

2. Trial of NO "ANTIDEPRESSANT" MEDICATION.

3. Add[103,104] or switch to a second MS (lithium, divalproex, carbamazepine, or lamotrigine, depending on mood state) or an AAP (**A**typical **A**nti**P**sychotic), thyroid augmentation, or psychotherapy.

4. Add (or switch to a different) AAP or a second or third MS, thyroid augmentation, psychotherapy, omega-3/fish oil, or adjunctive medication (e.g., zolpidem or eszopiclone or temazepam or other sedative-hypnotic for insomnia, or benzodiazepine or gabapentin for anxiety and/or insomnia).

5. Add (or switch to a different) AAP, third or fourth MS, Seroquel XR (quetiapine), olanzapine (Zyprexa), olanzapine-fluoxetine combination (OFC), thyroid augmentation, lurasidone (Latuda), psychotherapy, pramipexole, modafinil, omega-3/fish oil, unipolar AD (UAD/conventional AD), haloperidol or other older antipsychotic, or adjunctive medication (as in #4 above), or hospitalization with or without ECT (electro-convulsive treatment).

Now that we've described a general or generic template, we'll explain how it might be modified for different phases of the disorder.

B. **"DSM-IV-TR[24] Bipolar Depressive Episode;" and Depressive Mixed Episode (DMX):**

Please also refer to Chapter 5, "All Mixed Up," as, in my opinion, the widely used DSM-IV-TR[24] slices the pie in an unhelpful way. It gives way too small a slice of the pie to mixed episodes, and way too big a slice to what it calls bipolar depression.

The treatment of DMX may involve early use in the above sequential treatment model of the medicines likely to be effective for mixed episodes with a depressive flavor including lamotrigine, quetiapine, olanzapine, lithium, or possibly lurasidone or ziprasidone[218] (the bipolar ADs, or BADs[5,6,28,61,102,213,215,216,218]).

After 5 mood episodes or 5 to 10 years of illness, patients are in the late course of the disorder (Chapters 4 and 5), and only about 15% to 20% of patients presenting to a psychiatrist or other provider at that point are suffering from pure bipolar depression, as compared to about 40% of patients presenting with depressive mixed episode. Depressive mixed episode (DMX) might reasonably be expected to get worse with treatment with unipolar ADs.[13,68]

C. Pure Bipolar Depression

In the cycling-and-recurrence based bipolar treatment approach (CRBBT), patients are generally maintained on one or more of the traditional MSs (lithium, divalproex, carbamazepine, or lamotrigine), with or without an AAP, given in the absence of ADs. If the patient is either noted to have predominantly depressive episodes, or develops a pure bipolar depressive episode during the course of treatment, a cycling-and-recurrence based clinician would try to keep maintenance treatment and a long-term view in mind[33,43,143,190] while going through a mental checklist of the most likely effective options:

1. Has the patient had an adequate trial of lithium in the absence of ADs? Why lithium? Because, as described in Chapter 8 above, lithium provides mild to moderate protection against relapse into depression,[4,5,6,7,167,187,190,198] and lithium is the strongest anti-suicide medication known to man.[105,163-166]

2. Has the patient had an adequate trial of lamotrigine in the absence of AD medication? Lamotrigine deserves consideration, because it provides strong protection against relapse into bipolar depression.

3. Have we tried the AAP Seroquel XR/quetiapine XR at doses of 300 to 600 mg in the evening in the absence of ADs? This should be considered because it has demonstrated effectiveness and FDA approval for use in acute bipolar depression.

4. Have olanzapine (Zyprexa) or lurasidone been tried in the absence of

ADs? Olanzapine was until recently the only other AAP with demonstrated efficacy for acute bipolar depression.[102,213,214] It also has some evidence of protection against depressive relapse.[190]

Researchers have just very recently presented double-blind, placebo-controlled studies showing effectiveness of lurasidone (Latuda) in bipolar depression, either alone[213,215] or when added to lithium or divalproex.[213,216]

5. Has augmentation with thyroid medication been given an adequate trial? Studies have shown that patients with very, very mild hypothyroidism, or even normal circulating thyroid hormone levels with TSH values around 4 have a higher rate of depression (and possibly worse cycling) than patients with TSH values around 2.[144] TSH values at 2 and 4 are both entirely normal, but a value of 4 indicates just the tiniest bit less circulating thyroid hormone, and this seems to carry with it a vulnerability to bipolar depression. Very surprisingly also, as shown in Tables 9.1–9.4 below referring to the study by Post and others measuring treatment success rates in 525 bipolar patients, the addition of thyroid medication was the second or third most successful treatment intervention! Perhaps we should be considering this a bit more often.

6. Regardless of the medication treatments, we should certainly be considering psychotherapy, including those designed to restore the normal sleep-wake cycle and circadian rhythms (daily biological rhythms), and establish "lifestyle regularity," such as IPSRT (InterPersonal and Social Rhythms Therapy).[86,144,153] We might also include treatments that may be used as part of carefully designed strategies to re-establish the normal sleep-wake cycle, such as sleep deprivation and bright light therapy.

We might consider trying newer or alternative treatments, such as omega-3/fish oil (which has "strong evidence" for reduction of bipolar depressive symptoms[151]), or pramipexole.[195,196,197]

7. If none of the above have succeeded, one must consider more aggressive treatments, including the olanzapine-fluoxetine combination (OFC, Symbyax) which has demonstrated efficacy and FDA approval for the treatment of bipolar depression. Other more aggressive measures include psychiatric hospitalization, which needs to be considered at any point where the patient is at serious risk of self-harm or harm to others. Electro-convulsive treatment (ECT) is a powerful

and highly effective treatment for bipolar depression which would be considered in conjunction with hospitalization.[5,133]

8. Bear in mind that about 1 in 6 patients have been shown to maintain better long-term stability when a conventional AD medicine is included in their regimen, and if this is clearly demonstrated in a given patient, the AD should definitely be included. You can readily see, however, that there are several strategies with better success rates that might reasonably be considered before one considers adding an AD.

If the patient has been on the AD medicines for several months or a matter of years, and the patient still presents with ongoing serious mood episodes and a failure to reach stable recovery,[18,20] it may seem much less likely that the patient is one of the 1 in 6 bipolar patients who benefits long term from the ADs. One must then also consider the possibility that the ADs might be part of the problem, rather than part of the solution.[134]

After careful review and discussion, the patient and the treating clinician may in some cases decide to slowly and carefully taper and discontinue the ADs over a matter of several months. Once the mood episode is carefully characterized and a very gradual antidepressant taper is begun, the standard mood stabilizers start to have a better chance to work.

Even early in the process, many patients experience a distinct improvement in their mood stability, including, surprisingly enough, gradual but steady lessening of their depression.

During the process of tapering and discontinuing the ADs, the clinician and patient are patiently and systematically rotating through the 4 traditional MSs, with or without the AAPs, and various combinations of the above 2 classes of medicines if necessary. As my patients and I progress through this process, full major depressive episodes disappear altogether in about half of the patients, at the same time as the patients are on progressively lower doses of the conventional/unipolar ADs.[28,61]

If full pure major depressive episodes do still occur, one can then continue the MSs, with or without the AAPs, and sequentially and systematically rotate through the bipolar ADs[28,61] lamotrigine, quetiepine, lithium, olanzapine, and perhaps lurasidone.[5,6,28,61,102,190,213] One might certainly also consider thyroid augmentation or the olanzapine-fluoxetine combination, or possibly ziprasidone[218].

The specific use of the olanzapine-fluoxetine combination (OFC, Symbyax) has better proof of effectiveness than any of the unipolar antidepressants.[102,128]

Colleagues sometimes ask me what advantage the olanzapine-fluoxetine combination (OFC, Symbyax) has over any other combinations of AAP and AD. There are at least three:

1. We have convincing studies, leading to Food and Drug Administration (FDA) approval for marketing in the US, that OFC is effective for bipolar depression, and we have no convincing studies for bipolar depression for any of the many other potential combinations.

2. Olanzapine is one of only two or three AAPs that has demonstrated effectiveness against bipolar depression on its own, without combining it with any other medicine.[102,190,213,214] Quetiapine XR (Seroquel XR) is another. Very recent studies suggest that lurasidone (Latuda) may be the third.[213,215] The other newer antipsychotics have been tried, and thus far, the others have failed, aside from the use of ziprasidone to treat depressive mixed episode.[218]

3. From the Symbyax (olanzapine-fluoxetine combination/OFC) clinical trials, we have specific recorded data on the effectiveness, safety, and hazards of using these two medicines together in patients with bipolar disorder, and we don't have this data for any of the other numerous possible combinations.

If the patient has a history of a very positive initial response to one of the conventional ADs, the clinician might consider using this for 2-3 months (or less if it triggers worse cycling), followed by a very slow taper over several weeks or even a few months. If the conventional AD proves to be helpful longer-term and truly doesn't worsen cycling over the long term in this patient, the conventional AD probably should be continued in the medicine combination long-term.[10,15] A very visible notation should be made in the patient's chart, as we only observe this outcome in about 1 patient in 6, and this patient's treatment may be substantially different from that of most other patients.

There are a large number of treatments for bipolar depression other than conventional antidepressants. These treatments other than ADs are supported by varying amounts of evidence. Most of these are explained in the form of a case consultation, as described by Robert Post, M.D. and Gabriele Leverich, M.S.W., in Chapter 35 of *Treatment of Bipolar Illness, A Casebook for Clinicians and Patients*.[133]

D. Manic or Manic/Mixed Episode:

As noted above and in Chapter 5, "All Mixed Up," the widely used but narrowly-defined DSM-IV-TR[24] description gives mixed episodes too small a slice of the pie. Only about 5% or less of patients will arrive at the psychiatrist's office with a mixed episode that would meet the DSM-IV-TR[24] definition.

Instead, after 5 mood episodes or 5 to 10 years of illness, patients are in the late course of the disorder, and about 10% of patients presenting to a psychiatrist or other provider at that point will exhibit pure manic episode, and about 30% will present with a manic mixed episode (MMX), i.e., a mixed episode with a predominance of manic features.

Both these episode patterns will respond relatively well to the generic regimen shown in **A.** above, although to the extent that the patient has severe symptoms, difficulty with control, severe insomnia, etc., one may need to consider the possibility of hospitalization. One might also be inclined to start an AAP simultaneously with the primary MS immediately at the beginning of treatment, for more rapid clinical control.

E. Pure DSM-IV-TR[24] Mixed Episode:

Given how extremely demanding the criteria are (requiring both the full manic symptom cluster and the full depressive symptom pattern, almost every day for a week), this symptom pattern is likely to occur in only about 5% of real world bipolar patients. If one encounters this pure syndrome, it is likely to respond best to the initial strategy described in **A.** above. If, after successful control of manic and mixed symptoms, some depressive symptoms persist, then one should consider applying the strategies contained in **B.** above, which at that point might be successful. Unipolar ADs are, however, not likely to help, and may make this condition worse.[13,68]

A second approach to the treatment of bipolar disorder with which this chapter might be compared is Treatment As Usual in the community (TAU). As you will see, this provides a stark contrast to the sequential treatment model outlined above. TAU is usually a polarity-based treatment strategy (see Chapter 3). It seems to rely most heavily on use of the AD medications and, as a close second, on the antipsychotics (mostly the AAPs), both short-term and long-term.[8,9]

Very interestingly, TAU usually omits or avoids the treatments consistently demonstrated to be most effective in the long-term treatment of bipolar disorder, the traditional MSs. Many clinicians view traditional MSs as "toxic," or dangerous.

Indeed, there are some definite medical risks with the traditional MSs, although with proper training, clinicians can certainly learn how to deal with these associated risks, and monitor and manage these with the patients and their families quite safely.[1] Unfortunately these agents have largely been forgotten and have unreasonably fallen out of favor over the past 10 to 15 years, and therefore such training in how to use them is not widely available.

If one looks at the long term, the AAPs and ADs that treatment-as-usual clinicians prescribe instead are actually probably more risky than the MSs. The AAPs are associated with medical/"metabolic" side effects, such as weight gain, diabetes, and elevations of cholesterol and triglycerides. These changes may increase the risk of heart and blood vessel complications, such as heart attack and stroke. The AAPs also bring a small risk of an unwanted, lasting, and sometimes permanent movement disorder (tardive dyskinesia).

The antidepressants, on the other hand, have a very high likelihood of providing no improvement in the patient's condition. They are overall more likely to worsen the course of bipolar disorder than to improve it.[13,39,68] Worsening of the patient's bipolar disorder may lead to suicide, or much more commonly to loss of jobs, destruction of relationships, and inability to function in life, often for decades.

Aside from times of acute crises, effective bipolar regimens in the cycling and recurrence approach, by contrast, usually start with one of the traditional

---

1 Frederick Goodwin, M.D., may have may have described it most simply by describing one of the most effective mood stabilizers, and saying, in effect, "If you're not comfortable prescribing lithium, perhaps you shouldn't be treating bipolar disorder."[100]

"big three" mood stabilizers: lithium (Eskalith, LithoBID, and others), divalproex (Depakote, Depakote ER), or carbamazepine (Equetro, Tegretol, Carbatrol, and others).[5,6,98,99] In many patients with bipolar II disorder, the newest traditional MS, lamotrigine (Lamictal), may be a very reasonable starting place. One of the most important issues in the early treatment of the patient is finding which one of the traditional MSs is the most helpful and well-tolerated as the core of their regimen.

As with all medicines, the MSs also have their risks, for which the clinician must watch, and a partial listing of these follows.

Lithium requires following lithium blood levels and blood chemistries, as well as tests of kidney function and thyroid function. These can all be followed with periodic blood tests. Testing of kidney function may require testing the urine. Lithium use is not advised in patients with heart rhythm disorders, nor with diuretics, ACE inhibitor blood pressure medicines, or non-steroidal anti-inflammatory drugs (NSAIDs). Lithium is pregnancy class D, that is, it is associated with known birth defects. It is, however, probably the safest in pregnancy of the big three MSs.[148]

Divalproex requires following blood levels and blood tests of liver function. As with lithium and carbamazepine also, divalproex is pregnancy category D, that is, it is associated with a known risk of birth defects. Divalproex, however, has a somewhat higher risk of serious birth defects, such that it is not even recommended for women of childbearing age in Great Britain.[108] Divalproex also has a somewhat higher risk of weight gain than lithium or carbamazepine.

Carbamazepine has an approximately 1 in 1,000 risk of medically dangerous rash (much the same as the fourth mood stabilizer, lamotrigine/Lamictal), and this risk with carbamazepine appears to be greater in patients of South Asian ancestry. Carbamazepine is also pregnancy class D. Carbamazepine may interfere with the effectiveness of birth control pills, and patients taking birth control pills therefore need to discuss this with their OB/GYN specialists or other clinicians prescribing the birth control pills. It is important to follow blood levels of carbamazepine, the complete blood count, and certain chemistries, in particular sodium, in patients being treated with carbamazepine. On the other hand, carbamazepine is usually weight neutral.

Lamotrigine has the above-mentioned 1 in 1,000 risk of medically dangerous rash, but is usually weight neutral.

A recent study looked at various treatments and how many medicines the patient was taking in an attempt to control the bipolar disorder.[41] The researchers found that small, compact medication combinations contained one or more of the above "big three" traditional MSs, and the larger regimens contained ADs and antipsychotics,[41] the "bread and butter" of polarity-based treatment as usual.

One might certainly reason that if the early medications tried with a patient are effective, the clinician generally has to add fewer of them, but if the early medications are ineffective or possibly even make things worse, the clinician will find himself or herself feeling obliged to try adding other medications, thereby leading to a larger medication combination.[m] In this situation, however, it becomes hard to tell which medication, if any, is actually providing long-term benefit.

Since bipolar disorder is a long-term disorder, it might be very helpful to look at which medicines are successful in helping patients enter into stable periods of recovery for long periods of time.[18,20,143,190]

Fortunately, the Stanley Foundation Bipolar Network / Bipolar Collaborative Network group (SFBN/BCN, See Chapter 2) recently reported on a study of 525 bipolar outpatients followed for an average of 2.72 years, which looked at this very question.[20] They reported on the success rates of various medicines. The successful medicines, when started or added to the patients' medicine list, led to 6 months or more of substantial improvement. This sustained improvement of the responders was for an average of 17.8 months.

In Table 9.1 below, we find the observed success rates of medicines used in bipolar disorder, as listed in the above SFBN/BCN study.[20] In looking over Table 9.1 below, you'll see that clinicians operating from the cycling and recurrence approach are mostly using medicines #1, 2, 3, 4, 5, and 7 (newer antipsychotics), as shown in Table 9.1:

---

m Another feature of polarity-based treatment as usual is the tendency to keep adding medicines, rather than deciding that some of the medicines aren't helping, and replacing them (see Chapter 15). This results in regimens that keep getting bigger and bigger, but not necessarily better.

Success Rates of Various Medicine Subclasses and Individual Medicines
in Leading to Substantial Improvement for 6 Months or More
in a Large Naturalistic Clinical Trial[20]

Table 9.1, Cycling and Recurrence Approach

		Medicine Subclass or Individual Medicine:	Success Rate:
	1	Lithium	49.3%
	2	Carbamazepine	39.7%
	3	Thyroid Medicine (T3 or T4)	35.9%
	4	Divalproex/Valproate	34.8%
	5	Lamotrigine	24.8%
	6	SSRI Antidepressants	21.9%
(tie)	7	Newer Antipsychotics	20.7%
(tie)	7	Benzodiazepines	20.7%
(tie)	7	Trazodone	20.7%
	10	Bupropion	19.1%
	11	Topiramate	18.0%
	12	Gabapentin	17.0%
	13	Other Antidepressants	16.8%

We are now going to copy the exact same information from Table 9.1 above, and display it again as Table 9.2 below, but this time we will instead highlight from the same list the medicines most commonly prescribed by polarity-based clinicians, that is, medicines #6, 7 (newer antipsychotics, i.e., AAPs), 7 (trazodone), 10, and 13, as shown in grey color in Table 9.2.

Success Rates of Various Medicine Subclasses and Individual Medicines
in Leading to Substantial Improvement for 6 Months or More
in a Large Naturalistic Clinical Trial[20]

Table 9.2, Polarity-Based Approach

		Medicine Subclass or Individual Medicine:	Success Rate:
	1	Lithium	49.3%
	2	Carbamazepine	39.7%
	3	Thyroid Medicine (T3 or T4)	35.9%
	4	Divalproex/Valproate	34.8%
	5	Lamotrigine	24.8%
	6	SSRI Antidepressants	21.9%
(tie)	7	Newer Antipsychotics	20.7%
(tie)	7	Benzodiazepines	20.7%
(tie)	7	Trazodone	20.7%
	10	Bupropion	19.1%
	11	Topiramate	18.0%
	12	Gabapentin	17.0%
	13	Other Antidepressants	16.8%

As you can see from the first display of the table above, Table 9.1, Cycling and Recurrence Approach, the sequential treatment model strategy described earlier in this chapter was selected from the medicines with the highest success rates in leading to sustained recovery of 6 months or more.

Chapter 10

Tapering Antidepressants: More Art than Science

Remember, if you want to consider any changes to any aspect of your treatment, you need to discuss this with your own healthcare provider. Any potential changes need to be managed under their guidance and direction.

Clinical Case 10.1: Seemingly Surprising Clearing
of 30 Years of Depression

A woman in her mid-50s came to see me for one "last chance" consultation before giving up and consulting instead with the undertaker. She had been suffering depression since her 20s and been under psychiatric treatment with a number of psychiatrists since her early 30s, and had been given antidepressants and a host of other medications. She had been hospitalized a number of times without much lasting benefit.

In her mid-40s, her diagnosis was changed from major depression to bipolar disorder, and her successive doctors tried adding various mood stabilizers, and some potential mood stabilizers such as Topamax/topirimate, to her regimen of antidepressants and antipsychotics, but her doctors never in the course of her treatment of over 25 years tried mood stabilizer treatment without antidepressants.

She came to me totally discouraged and hopeless. When she was asked her symptoms directly and in detail, she reported both severe manic and severe depressive symptoms. That is, she was in the midst of a relatively severe bipolar mixed episode.[24] When asked her complete lifetime history of mood episodes in detail, she described at least two fairly convincing hypomanic episodes (small manias)[24] in her late teens, which her other doctors had apparently not asked about or discovered. That is, her bipolar disorder had actually first begun in her teens, but, as very often happens, this wasn't diagnosed until many years later.[58, 63-66,146,201,202]

She then had more serious manic episodes in her 40s leading to the eventual change in diagnosis to bipolar disorder. She was on disability and convinced she was a hopeless case, and that nothing could be done for her, but she came anyway, almost against hope. On her arrival at the initial interview, she was on seven psychiatric medications, including two conventional antidepressants.

One of my initial impulses was to remove most of the seven psychiatric medications she was taking, as her medication regimen appeared somewhat over-complicated and mysterious. After discussing this in some detail with the patient, however, we decided instead on a different sort of clinical experiment.

Patients with late course bipolar disorder, that is, several mood episodes or several years into the illness (and this patient had over 35 years of bipolar illness), generally describe the same symptoms this patient described, i.e., rapid cycling or worse,[n] mixed episodes, and much more conscious experience of the symptoms as "depression" (see also Chapters 4 and 5).

It is interesting that they tend to describe this as "depression" rather than "mania," as they usually also report (when asked) serious insomnia, irritability, racing thoughts, distractibility, impulsivity, edginess, and anxiety. That is, they are also experiencing quite a few symptoms of over-activation, i.e., significant manic symptoms as part of a mixed state.

The only medication interventions that have seemed to help in my experience with patients in the late course of bipolar disorder are: 1. the addition of mood stabilizers, and 2. the taper and removal of conventional antidepressants. Overall, in the majority of such cases, the removal of antidepressant medication

---

n Rapid cycling[24] refers to bipolar illness with 4 or more total mood episodes per year. Many patients in the late course, however, suffer even more frequent cycling. They may have ultra-rapid cycling (4 or more episodes in a week), 'ultradian' cycling (with multiple episodes occurring in the same day), or perhaps even more commonly, rapidly shifting mixed episodes (Figure 4.4).

has seemed to be absolutely necessary for success.

The patient and I therefore essentially decided not to touch any of her other medications, but just spend the next several months tapering the two antidepressants, as I had seen again and again that most of my bipolar patients seemed to do better without them if we could succeed in removing them.

Removing them had proved to be tricky in these prior patients, however, and seemed to work best when done very, very slowly and patiently, over a span of 8 to 12 months, especially if they had been on antidepressants for years.

It also required explaining the ultimate goal to the patient (of getting off the antidepressants altogether), and also alerting them that they might well experience some down or other somewhat upsetting feelings for the first 5 to 10 days after each dose reduction. I explain that many of these symptoms are actually only mild withdrawal symptoms and that they will pass, often during the first week. Just knowing where we were going and what to expect has made the patients much more comfortable with the process.

So, getting back to our case, we left all the other medications in my patient's regimen, and just very gradually tapered the two antidepressants over the next 11 months. She encountered no major difficulty with this, and in fact showed some slow, steady improvement, with steady, gradual reduction of reported depression and anxiety over this time, and a gradually increasing sense of calm.

By the time of her first office visit after getting off the antidepressants completely, she had gone from her initial very fretful, nervous, extremely discouraged state to being extremely calm, relaxed, and with a very easy smile I had never seen with her before. She had no sense of any depression whatsoever. All of her manic and depressive symptoms had gone from the severe range to the minimal range, or had cleared completely.

Although I was again tempted to remove some of her medicines because of the seemingly unnecessarily large medicine list, I decided to just leave everything the same, without the antidepressants, and for the next 19 months, she remained entirely free of mood episodes, a situation she had never experienced before in her 30 years of prior treatment.

We then tried to reduce one of her two antipsychotic medications because of a potential drug interaction. She then started to experience manic symptoms, but called my office promptly. We resumed her prior higher and more effective antipsychotic medicine dose, with rapid clearing of the manic symptoms. She then returned to stable moods with no major mood episodes for several months thereafter.

As yet there are no studies and almost no guidance as to how to do tapering and removal of antidepressant medications in bipolar patients. This would seem quite surprising, given that this seems to be one of the most important changes needed.

When one looks up the topic of antidepressant taper, one finds information about how to reduce antidepressants over several days to a couple of weeks so as to avoid SSRI (selective serotonin reuptake inhibitor) withdrawal syndrome, which involves feeling spacey, foggy, dizzy, weak, and jittery, with possible headache, nausea, vomiting, or diarrhea, if one goes off the very popular SSRI or SNRI (selective serotonin and norepinephrine reuptake inhibitor) antidepressants "cold turkey."[132] One might also find a couple of case reports or papers on abrupt antidepressant removal triggering manic episodes in bipolar patients.[192,193] However, as one recent article notes, "Tapering antidepressants is more art than science because we have no controlled data to support any particular tapering regimen."[132]

At least one bipolar expert recommends somewhat more gradual taper of antidepressants over weeks to months for bipolar patients.[107] In my experience, trying to taper bipolar patients off the antidepressants over a matter of weeks seems to lead to the patient re-experiencing feelings of bad mood described and experienced by the patient as "depression," especially if the patient has been on antidepressants for years. If, however, I alert the patient to the possibility of a few days of generally manageable and very temporary bad feelings with each dose reduction, and then taper the medication very slowly over several months, we often succeed at getting them off the antidepressant medication altogether. Occasionally, as in Clinical Cases 15.2 and 17.1, more rapid tapers may be successful.

In a smaller number of cases, we find that the patient is probably one of the 1 in 6 patients who does better remaining on some antidepressant medication, but they are often nonetheless somewhat calmer and more stable on a lower dose of the antidepressant medication than they had been taking before. For those who seem to do significantly better on their full prior dose of antidepressant medicine, we simply take note of that and continue them on it for as long as that continues to work best for them.

When I raised this topic with bipolar disorder experts at the International Conference of the International Society for Bipolar Disorders in Pittsburgh, in June 2011, none saw any objection to tapering antidepressant medications in bipolar patients over intervals as long as 6 to 12 months, especially if the patient has been taking antidepressants for several months or for a matter of years. This is the strategy that I have found to work best for my own patients over the past few years. Systematic study in this area would be welcome, and might provide us clues and guidance to greater success.

CALM SEAS

Section C:

Key Treatment Relationship Issues

Chapter 11

Discovering Each Patient's Lifetime History of Mood Disorders

Forming a strong treatment relationship with the patient (and, where appropriate, with their family or close support person[s]), beginning with the first session, is as important with bipolar disorder as it is with any other treatment in psychiatry. Without it, diagnosis is less likely to be accurate, and treatment is more likely to fail.

Unless the patient comes with a clear and convincing diagnosis of bipolar disorder, it is important to start the interview with a professional but warm demeanor, and with a very broad focus to one's listening, e.g., "How may I help?" or "Please tell me what's bothering you."

As the patient is telling his or her story, the clinician is listening carefully **vertically** or **top-down** (as to the severity and urgency of the disorder), and how the disorder unfolds over time. One is also listening carefully to the nature of the symptoms, and also listening between related classes of disorders, to see which class of disorders fits best with the condition the patient is describing.

It gradually becomes clear what class of disorder the patient may suffer, for instance, mood disorder vs. psychotic disorder vs. personality disorder vs. anxiety disorder vs. cognitive (thinking) disorder. Once this is discovered (not always within the first session or two), the clinician is listening within classes, to see if the pattern of a specific disorder fits tightly.

To the extent possible, it is best to let the patient tell his or her story without much interruption. If, however, the patient is complaining about a significant, very disruptive mood disorder, and the broad initial story they give supports this, then their current situational everyday upsets may not be as important as finding out both their recent mood symptoms and a full lifetime history of mood episodes, from the beginning of the first major mood symptoms.

Often these have started in childhood or adolescence. Without hearing and recording and understanding the full lifetime mood history, the current mood symptoms may be misinterpreted and the mood disorder may be diagnosed incorrectly.

Now some doctors might feel that trying to get the mood history fairly early might involve steering and directing the interview too much, as opposed to listening in considerable detail to the patient's current life struggles.

On the other hand, a first interview with the psychiatrist is not altogether unlike the oral examination of the psychiatry board certification exam of the American Board of Psychiatry and Neurology.

In this examination, a candidate psychiatrist would interview a psychiatric patient in the presence of two senior psychiatrist examiners. If the interviewing psychiatrist missed the presence of a potentially disabling or life-threatening severe psychiatric disorder, such as organic brain syndrome, uncontrolled active drug or alcohol addiction, schizophrenia, or bipolar disorder (see Chapter 12), the interviewing psychiatrist would likely fail the exam. If one misses any of these urgent disorders in one's clinical practice, one is likely to fail to provide reasonable care for the patient.

Part of the reason some doctors might have concerns about finding out the full mood history during the first session or two is that this might be perceived as a failure of hearing the patient's concerns. Thus, the approach I describe here is more clearly warranted if the patient identifies mood episodes as a major source of their distress. If they do so, then not to explore the mood episodes throughout their lifetime might be the greater failure of understanding.

Patients are very clear in describing their perception of whether their clinicians, including their psychiatrists over the years, understand the nature of their emotional struggles. For this reason, I am very direct in asking my patients to correct me if I am misunderstanding what they are explaining to me. I point out to them, and to their closest support person if present, that I am only just getting to know them. They have a lot to explain and describe to me, so that I can better understand the nature of their distress and concerns.

Chapter 12

Top-Down View:
The Rarely-Discussed, but
Absolutely Essential Topic
of Hierarchic Diagnosis
(Diagnosis by Rank Order)

Case 12.1

A young woman in her 20s, supposedly attending college, but seemingly more preoccupied with the night life on campus, came to see a psychiatrist after 4 failed antidepressant trials, and asked the psychiatrist to help her try yet another antidepressant.

A reasonably detailed history of mood episodes and current mood symptoms clearly indicated that if the patient did have a primary mood disorder separate from her alcohol abuse, that it was bipolar disorder rather than major depressive disorder. (Active alcohol or drug abuse makes it hard to diagnose anything else, however, including mood disorders.)

The patient showed no real interest in the psychiatrist's questioning as to whether she might consider sobriety and beginning active recovery with Alcoholics Anonymous. As you'll see below, without successful treatment of the more urgent alcohol abuse and likely bipolar disorder, attempts to treat the depressive symptoms would be doomed to fail.

An important aspect of understanding the mood disorders, and bipolar disorder in particular, is the importance of hierarchic diagnosis, that is, diagnosis by urgency and rank order, i.e., **top-down**. Some disorders are more urgent to identify first, and if one fails to do so, one misses the opening to successful treatment.

In a moment we will get to a table showing where the various psychiatric disorders fit in this rank ordering, but first, one might certainly wonder why this is so important, and five factors come immediately to mind:

1. Urgency
2. Mimicry
3. The Potential to Worsen the Course of the Disorder
4. Likely Treatment Failure
5. Strong Family History, Suggesting a Major Genetic Component to the Disorder

The following section explains the above factors in more detail:

1. Urgency. Certain disorders are generally more severe and time-sensitive than others, and thus need to be considered first. Some of this thinking flows from an ER mind-set.[119] The emergency room doctor and staff are very concerned with disorders with a high likelihood of killing the patient in 30 minutes (and thus possibly before the ER doctor and staff can save them). They are less urgently concerned with disorders that have a high or moderate likelihood of killing the patient in 30 weeks, for instance, because the patient is much more likely to leave the ER and the hospital alive and be in a position to be cared for successfully by their primary doctor and/or specialists as an outpatient.

This urgency item originally began during the writing of this chapter as "Severity," and tier 1 disorders are overall, as a group, more severe than tier 2 disorders, but there are important exceptions. For instance, bipolar disorders are tier 1 disorders and are overall more severe than the tier 2 major depressive disorders (unipolar depressions).[158] However, some unipolar major depressions are quite severe, with considerable suicide risk.[o] If severity alone were the way of deciding, one could easily argue that these severe major depressions should be relabeled as tier 1 disorders.

---

o The same is also true for many severe cases of PTSD, although, as an anxiety disorder, this would be listed in this system as a tier 2 disorder.

In contrast to severity alone, however, urgency incorporates Items 2, 3, and 4 below, whereas severity alone does not. It thus became clear that urgency is a better way to explain this, including the whole idea of hierarchic diagnosis. As in Case 12.1 above, and as will be explained below, when a mood disorder is present it is much more urgent to determine whether it is a bipolar disorder than whether major depression is present.

2. Mimicry. This refers to the ability of one disorder to fool us into thinking it is another disorder. In hierarchic diagnosis, mimicry occurs only in one direction, **downward mimicry**. For example, bipolar disorders can and frequently do mimic major depressive disorders. Major depressive disorders cannot, however, mimic bipolar disorders, as manias and mixed states never occur in major depressive disorders, by DSM-IV-TR definition.[24] If they do, according to DSM-III,[120] DSM-IV,[11] and DSM-IV-TR,[24] the condition is automatically re-classified as bipolar disorder, because one of the defining features of major depressive disorder is that it is a uni-polar disorder. That is, mood swings only go in 1 direction, down, into depression. If the mood swings of the condition ever go in 2 directions, it is by definition a bi-polar disorder.[11,24,155] Bipolar disorders include not only down mood swings, but also up (manic and mixed) mood swings.

Put another way, bipolar disorders exhibit all the necessary features to qualify for the diagnosis of major depressive disorder, that is, depressive episodes. On the other hand, major depressive disorders do not have all the clinical features to be diagnosed as bipolar disorder, that is, they do not exhibit manic or mixed episodes. Upward mimicry is not possible in this system.

When major depressive disorder seems to be mimicking bipolar disorder, it is usually a wake-up call to all involved to re-evaluate the condition, as this usually signals that the disorder is indeed bipolar disorder rather than unipolar disorder.

3. The potential to worsen the course of the disorder. The third reason for diagnosing according to a hierarchy, or a top-down rank order system, is the possibility of specific treatments or treatment changes causing worsening of the clinical course of the condition. For instance, mood stabilizers have no inherent ability to worsen the course of unipolar disorder, but unipolar antidepressants[28,61]

(conventional or standard antidepressants) do have the potential to cause considerable worsening of bipolar disorder.[12,13,25,26,27,37] In a conference in the 1980s, therefore, Steven Dubovsky, M.D., then chairman of psychiatry at the University of Colorado, recommended that if there was significant doubt about whether a disorder was unipolar (major depression) or bipolar, that one might be well advised to consider starting a mood stabilizer rather than an antidepressant.

4. Likely treatment failure. Fourth, and related in part to Item 3, which we just discussed, is the issue of likely treatment failure. Ignoring hierarchic diagnosis leads very predictably to treatment failure. Consider the following clinical case:

Case 12.2

A man was seen at a public clinic in his late 20s and diagnosed with bipolar disorder. A number of doctors who saw him there over the years agreed on this diagnosis, and he was eventually successfully stabilized on a medication regimen including the mood stabilizer Depakote (divalproex) and the atypical antipsychotic Clozaril (clozapine) and functioned significantly better for a couple of years.

He then moved to a different city and enrolled in a public clinic there. The doctor who saw him there concluded from a single interview that instead of a primary diagnosis of bipolar disorder, he suffered post-traumatic stress disorder (PTSD), and had made "some bad choices" with his life. (He had indeed suffered some trauma, and, as almost all bipolar patients, he had made some bad life choices, and readily admitted these. Bipolar patients can certainly also suffer PTSD, but this needs to be addressed after the top tier disorder, the bipolar disorder, is controlled.)

The new doctor, however, then proceeded to dismantle the patient's prior successful bipolar disorder regimen and put him on different medicines more suitable for his new primary diagnosis of PTSD, that is, SSRI antidepressants. Over the next year his condition worsened considerably, but this didn't seem to concern his new doctor, who continued full speed ahead treating him for PTSD, and ignoring the prior tier 1 diagnosis of bipolar disorder.

The patient was very frustrated at getting worse, especially since he had previously been doing much better on the regimen for bipolar disorder. He therefore eventually found his way to a private psychiatrist, who carefully re-evaluated him and considered top-tier (tier 1) disorders first. This led him to confirm the prior primary diagnosis of bipolar disorder, and to shift the patient back to his prior bipolar medicine regimen, with significant improvement in his condition.

If a top-tier disorder is present (such as bipolar disorder), one must recognize it first, and control it first with treatment. If one fails to do so, then efforts at treating lower tier disorders (including major depressive disorder) first will almost always fail. This comes full circle to the ER mentality[119] pointed out above in the first issue of urgency:

Case 12.3

If an ER patient is bleeding very rapidly from a gaping wound, then ignoring the wound and the bleeding, and instead focusing completely on trying to manage the patient's anxiety is likely to fail.

Another example of this is given in Case 15.2, in Chapter 15. The hospital team apparently ignored the chance to control more aggressively first the top-tier bipolar I disorder, manic type. Instead, they focused their attention on treating the second-tier anxiety disorder, obsessive-compulsive disorder (OCD). They added an SSRI antidepressant, which could have helped the OCD, but which might have been expected to worsen the bipolar disorder. By the next night the patient didn't sleep (that is, she started to have much worse [top-tier] bipolar mania).

To translate this into the ER example (Case 12.3) above, it was as if they had focused on the ER patient's anxiety first, but in the process ignored and worsened the serious bleeding.

5. Strong Family History, Suggesting a Major Genetic Component to the Disorder. Finally, the disorders in tier 1 have the strongest family histories of the

disorder, and thus are more likely to be inherited. That is, these are more likely to be biologic diseases or illnesses caused in part by genetic factors, rather than just clusters of symptoms often found together, which might not be biologic illnesses at all. Definite biologic illnesses are felt to be likely somewhat more serious and thereby more urgent than mere clusters of symptoms of uncertain origin.

Some tier 2 disorders, including major depressive disorder (unipolar disorder) do have family history and genetic factors, and are also likely biologic disorders. Bipolar disorder, however, is more strongly linked to a positive family history and genetic factors than tier 2 disorders, including major depressive disorder.

We'll now move on to a graphic display of hierarchic diagnosis, to see visually where these conditions fit, in Table 12.1:

Table 12.1

Hierarchic Diagnosis					
TOP TIER	Medical or Neurologic Brain Disorders, "OBS, Organic Brain Syndrome"	Schizophrenia	Bipolar Disorders	Substance Abuse Disorders	Severe Anorexia Nervosa
2nd TIER	Milder Cognitive (Thinking) Problems, ADHD, Sleep Disorders	Milder Paranoid Disorders, Anxiety Disorders, Trauma Disorders	Unipolar Disorders (Serious Depressions Without Manias)	Anxiety Disorders and Trauma Disorders	Other Eating Disorders, Body Dysmorphic Disorder
3rd TIER	Vague Memory Complaints, or Vague, Neurologic-Sounding Complaints	Milder Suspiciousness or Anxiety Neurotic Disorders Personality Disorders	Mild, or Mild-to-Moderate Depression Adjustment Disorders, Relationship Difficulties	Diffuse Bodily and Pain Complaints Personality Disorders	Vague or Mild Concerns About Body Image

You'll readily see that all the top tier disorders can kill a lot of patients, whether treated or not. Four of the top tier disorders are relatively common:

1. Medical or Neurologic Brain Disorders (Organic Brain Syndrome)
2. Alcohol and Drug Addictions (Substance Use Disorders)
3. Schizophrenia
4. Bipolar Disorder

These distinctions between tiers are based in part on relative overall urgency of the condition. The second-tier disorders are overall not quite as urgent as the top-tier disorders, but are all also clearly disorders and many are probably disease states (medical and biochemical illnesses). By contrast, the third-tier conditions are generally not diseases, and some of them are not even distinct, treatable conditions.

To some, this hierarchic, top-down diagnosis idea will seem radical, but on this one, even the American Psychiatric Association *Diagnostic and Statistical Manuals* specify and require this kind of hierarchic diagnosis, and have consistently done so for the past 33 years since the first printing of DSM-III[120] in 1980.

This pecking order is explained in the above manuals by what are called "exclusion criteria." For instance, major depressive disorder **simply cannot be diagnosed** unless DSM-IV-TR's Criterion C is met: "There has never been a Manic Episode (see p. 169), a Mixed Episode (see p. 171), or a Hypomanic Episode (see p. 171)"[24] unless these are caused by street drugs, medical treaments (such as unipolar antidepressants, steroids, or ECT), or directly caused by a general medical condition.[24] That is, according to the standard Diagnostic and Statistical Manual, and as clearly as can possibly be stated, if there is clear evidence of bipolar disorder, the diagnosis is bipolar disorder. In this case, the diagnosis of major depressive disorder (unipolar depression) is rejected by DSM-IV-TR,[24] and simply cannot be applied.

So you can immediately see that this way of organizing diagnoses has been present since 1980; it is nothing new. It has, however, often been largely forgotten or ignored or denied in the current clinical approach to the everyday treatment of patients suffering mood disorders. One example of this would be when an accurately-diagnosed bipolar patient is suddenly told by a new clinician that they now have major depressive disorder (unipolar disorder) instead. If the original bipolar disorder diagnosis was accurate, then such a change in a patient's diagnosis simply cannot occur.

In summary, it is important to ferret out any top-tier disorders such as bipolar disorder first, and treat them to a point of stable recovery. Other conditions lower on the hierarchy simply cannot be diagnosed accurately and with reasonable confidence until this happens. Once the top-tier disorder(s) is (are) treated to stable recovery, one then looks to see if the lower-tier disorders even persist. Often they do not. If they do persist, then we would look at how to treat them without worsening the top-tier disorders.

In summary, bipolar disorder can mimic and mistakenly be thought to be other lesser disorders, in particular, major depression,[23,58,63,64,65,94,140] thereby putting the bipolar patient at considerable hazard while they're being treated with strategies more likely to worsen their primary condition than improve it.

Chapter 13

Some Clinical Approaches for Bipolar I and II Patients, Including Listening, Collaboration, and Victory Laps

We'll start with a patient with a relatively solid and easily confirmed diagnosis of bipolar I or bipolar II disorder.   The description of the collaborative care model[30] was chosen as our starting place with such patients. I was describing it briefly to one of the psychiatric residents[p] I met at the 9th International Conference of the International Society for Bipolar Disorders in 2011. She immediately lit up with considerable interest. I therefore suspected it would also be of high interest to patients, families, and possibly to other clinicians.

The collaborative care model has perhaps been most completely described by Gary Sachs, M.D., of the Massachusetts General Hospital bipolar disorders program.[30] The model has some similarities to strategies used for years by some thoughtful internal medicine doctors to rehabilitate their patients with chronic diseases such as asthma and diabetes.

(Please note that if the patient were not suffering bipolar disorder, and instead suffered with recurrent unsuccessful behavior patterns rooted in childhood traumas or conflicts, or were suffering primarily with symptoms related to emotional trauma, a more traditional 1:1 therapy approach with few or no outside

p See Glossary for description of psychiatric residents.

inputs might be much more helpful and effective.)

I meet with the patient suffering with bipolar disorder, and if possible sooner rather than later with the patient together with their one closest and trusted support person (spouse, family member, very close and supportive friend, etc.).[4,6,7,159] The support person's history is valuable in confirming, rejecting, or modifying the diagnosis, and their collaboration in developing a realistic and workable treatment plan is also extremely helpful.

I start by explaining that in order for the patient to experience steadier moods and eventually to function better, that he/she and his/her support person will need to become experts in understanding the disorder, and that it is an important part of my job to teach them whatever they need to know.

I ask if either of them is a reader, and if so, I give them some selected references and websites to start learning about the disorder and its treatment, including copies of one or both of my overview letters to the editor (written together with S. Nassir Ghaemi, M.D., M.P.H., see the following references). As soon as it's available, I'll be giving them a copy of this book.

Recommended References for Patients and their Families:
- *Why Am I Still Depressed?* 2006, by Jim Phelps, M.D., a bipolar specialist in Oregon.
- CALM (Sparhawk and Ghaemi, 2008[33]).
- Depression and Bipolar Support Alliance (DBSA) website: www. dbsalliance.org
- Jim Phelps' website: www.psycheducation.org
- Jamison, Kay Redfield, 1995. *An Unquiet Mind.* New York, NY: Vintage Books.
- CALM SEA (Sparhawk and Ghaemi, 2011[43]).
- Sparhawk (2013), *CALM SEAS, Keys to the Successful Treatment of Bipolar Disorder.* CreateSpace, an Amazon Company.
- Our website: www.calmseas.us

I then start by explaining to them that bipolar disorder is a disorder of cycling, that is, increasing and decreasing levels of mood and energy, or **activation** (see Chapter 16). I further explain that in order to control the patient's symptoms and improve his/her functioning, that we must calm the cycling. I show them a very simplified cycle chart depicting a manic episode, a depressive episode, a simple mixed episode, and a rapidly-shifting mixed episode (See Figure 13.1).

Figure 13.1

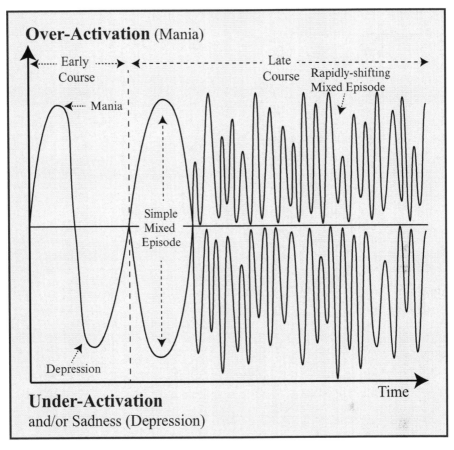

I point out to them that the most costly and high-risk parts of the disorder are often the extreme parts of the manic spells, during which they are likely to act impulsively and burn their bridges. The extreme parts of the depressive spells (Figure 13.2) are also very costly. During the extreme pure depressive spells, patients may sleep 10-20 hours per 24 hours and essentially be unable to do anything at all.

Figure 13.2

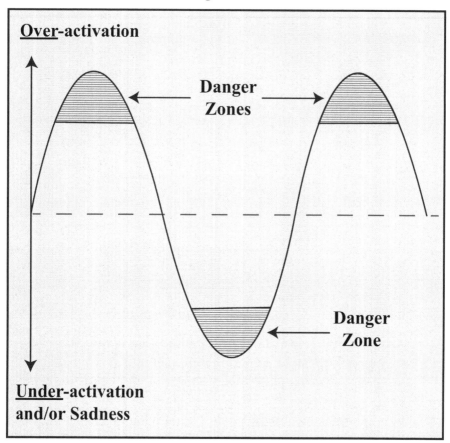

I then show them a second smoother curve (Figure 13.3) superimposed on the first mood episode diagram, and explain to them that we need to contain the extreme swings and compress them toward the horizontal midline. We also need to try to slow the swings, such that the swings occur less frequently and more gradually.

Figure 13.3

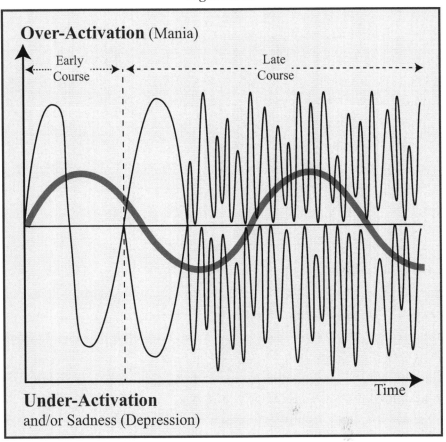

I paint for them the visual image of the surface of a pond (to mimic the horizontal midline), and explain that our goal is to keep the surface of the pond smooth. This helps them to begin to understand why more gradual changes to the treatment, including more gradual medication changes, may often work much better. I also give them a verbal image for this, CALM SEAS, and the corresponding earlier letter to the editor (CALM SEA[43], see also Chapter 7), which use this as a memory device to summarize the major treatment considerations regarding medication treatment and essential lifestyle modifications.

While working with patients and their families, the cycling-and-recurrence based clinician is usually addressing a number of issues listed below as A and B, 1 through 3:

A. Listening. Listening is the most important job when caring for any patient. The bipolar specialist has to be listening 100% of the time to the words and non-verbal messages of patients with bipolar disorder. When their families are present, the doctor needs to be listening carefully to them also. The specialist may have an advantage in understanding many of these messages from the patient and family, because of a more complete understanding of what they may be going through with the disorder. The clinician must nonetheless constantly be alert to hear new information, surprises, and new material, which may force the clinician to completely rethink his or her conception of the patient's disorder and overall condition.

B. While listening full-time as described above, there are various other tasks with patients with a solid diagnosis of bipolar I or bipolar II disorder. The clinician's remaining efforts are split in large part between three other everyday tasks.

1. The first of these is adding or adjusting traditional mood stabilizers. Many patients are treated instead with antidepressants, antipsychotics, anti-restlessness medicines, anti-anxiety medicines, sleep medicines, ADHD medicines, and occasionally, lamotrigine (Lamictal) or other mood stabilizers.

The three mood stabilizers most often not tried and/or left out are lithium, divalproex, and carbamazepine,[112,129] which coincidentally happen to be three of the medicines most convincingly shown to be effective in bipolar disorder over the long term.[20,21,41,103,104,111,116,187]

Lamotrigine appears to have had a rush of recent popularity. The scientific evidence would suggest that lamotrigine be used in place of conventional antidepressants, but curiously, it is instead often being paired with them, which then provides only a weak anti-manic ceiling to counter the unstable upward push of the antidepressants.

2. The second task which shares time with listening is discussing at length with patients and their families the antidepressant medicines that the vast

majority of bipolar patients have been taking long-term when they first come to see me, usually without benefit. If the patient and family are willing, and with adequate explanation, they usually are, we then start tapering the antidepressant medicines in those who do not believe they have had lasting benefit from these medicines (See Chapter 10).

3. The third, and fortunately fairly common and quite enjoyable task that comes up if we proceed in a careful and orderly fashion through Items A, B1, and B2, above, is that of victory laps. The patients come in dramatically calmer, with the prior considerable tension gone from their faces. When family members or support people come along, they are just floored at the change. The patients are very relaxed, often more so than they have been in years. They also have much improved daytime energy, interest, motivation, concentration, enjoyment, and confidence. They are now more able and more likely to complete tasks, and even take on activities they haven't done in years. Sleep is now more consistent, of normal duration, and of much better quality. They wake up rested. They appear calm, radiant, and beaming. Thinking and speech have returned to normal rates.

Some of them will comment, "This must be how normal is supposed to feel." They may then develop a questioning look on their faces and ask something to the effect of, "How do you do normal?" For many patients, it has been so long since they felt normal that they're a little uneasy and unsure as to how to go about this.

We take some time to savor and enjoy the dramatic improvement, and then we start to explore and develop some of the answers to the patients' question of "How do you do normal?

When patients finally reach stable recovery, they are indeed a little baffled. They think this was what they wanted, but when they get there, they're not sure how they should deal with it.

It is important for the doctor and family to understand that although this is a good change, it is still a very different way of experiencing the world and their life. Patients may need a bit of help adjusting to this change. Just telling the patient that you understand that they might feel somewhat disoriented for a while may be helpful to them. They can then begin to understand that this change is a normal part of the process of getting well.

Further Reading for healthcare professionals:

- Sachs, Gary, 2004. *Managing Bipolar Affective Disorder*. London, UK: Science Press. Chapter 1: Introduction to the Collaborative Care Model, pp. 1-22.
- Ghaemi, S. Nassir, 2008. *Mood Disorders*, *2nd Ed*. Practical Guides in Psychiatry. Philadelphia, PA: Wolters Kluwer Health.
- *Why Am I Still Depressed?* 2006, by Jim Phelps, M.D., a bipolar specialist in Oregon.
- Jamison, Kay Redfield, 1995. *An Unquiet Mind*. New York, NY: Vintage Books.
- Goodwin, Frederick K., and Jamison, Kay Redfield, 2007. *Manic-Depressive Illness: Bipolar Disorders and Recurrent Depression, 2nd Edition*. Oxford, UK: Oxford University Press.
- Post, Robert M., and Leverich, Gabriele S., 2008. *Treatment of Bipolar Illness: A Casebook for Clinicians and Patients*. New York, NY: W. W. Norton & Company.
- Sachs GS, Nierenberg AA, Calabrese JR, et al. Effectiveness of adjunctive antidepressant treatment for bipolar depression. N Engl J Med 2007; 356(17):1711-1722.
- Post RM, Altshuler LL, Frye MA, et al. Complexity of pharmacologic treatment required for sustained improvement in outpatients with bipolar disorder. Journal of Clinical Psychiatry 2010; 71(9):1176-1186.
- Post RM, Leverich GS, Altshuler LL, et al. Differential clinical characteristics, medication usage, and treatment response in the US versus The Netherlands and Germany. Intl Clin Psychopharmacol 2011; 26(2):96-106.
- Goldberg JF, Brooks JO, Kutita K, et al. Depressive Illness Burden Associated with Complex Polypharmacy in Patients with Bipolar Disorder: Findings from the STEP-BD. J Clin Psychiatry 2009;70(2):155-162.

Chapter 14

"Copping Some Attitudes" To Achieve More Complete and Sustained Recovery:

Greedy, Stubborn, Stingy, and the Dan Morgan Mentality of the Battle of Cowpens

When I did my medical training years ago (prior to my psychiatry specialty training), it was standard practice to predict poor outcomes for patients and their families. This was described as "Hanging the Crepe." It was reasoned back then that if you painted a somewhat bleak picture, and a bad outcome did occur, the patient and family would be prepared rather than surprised. If, on the other hand, the patient did well, the patient and family would be very pleasantly surprised.

Over the next several years, and for a number of reasons, I have arrived at just the opposite approach to predicting outcomes. I point out to patients and their families that bipolar disorder itself is extremely treatable. I tell them that we should expect a good outcome for the bipolar disorder, and that none of us should be happy about the situation until we get it.

Our clinical work is all about patient outcomes, and outcomes are strongly influenced by attitudes. Therefore, in one of the first few sessions, I often ask new patients with bipolar I or II disorder if anyone has ever told them they're stubborn. Many say yes. Some say this a bit sheepishly. I then ask them if anyone ever told them that their stubbornness was a good thing, and many say no, so I tell them, "Well then, let me be the first to do so!"

For the patients who say no one has ever told them they're stubborn, I tell them, "Don't worry, we'll teach you." The reason stubbornness is so important is that bipolar disorder is a top-tier disorder (one of the most serious disorders, see Chapter 12), and the recovery from any top-tier disorder is difficult and requires staying power, persistence, or stubbornness, however you like to put it.

Now that I've stimulated their interest a bit, I go on to admit to my patients that I'm also greedy. That is, I'm greedy for a good outcome for them, and they should be too. They are by then not totally surprised when I admit to them that I'm also stingy, and they should be too.

In summary, I tell them that we need to be greedy for a good result. This means stable recovery, that is, at least 2 to 6 months with no major mood episodes.[18,20] It is important that this also involve substantial gradual improvement in the patient's ability to function,[210] which it usually does. We then work hard to maintain this stability for several months or years.

We need to be stubborn in pursuing and achieving the good result. It is also important to be stingy in doing so with as little risk as possible, while still insisting on the good result.

I sometimes discuss with the patients and their families the Cowpens mentality, but I operate with it with every bipolar patient:

In early 1781 during the American Revolution, General Dan Morgan, with 600 American troops, was being chased across South Carolina by Lieutenant Colonel Banastre Tarleton, a cavalry officer deservedly known as "The Butcher," with 1,100 British soldiers.[109] Rather than trying to escape them, Morgan was looking for an advantageous place to fight them. He chose the Cowpens, where his men would have the advantage of facing the British from behind two low hills overlooking the pasture through which the British would be approaching them.

On the other hand, to the Americans' backs was "a deep stream that would cut off all escape if Morgan and his men were beaten."[109] In essence, every American soldier on the field that day could see that if they were beaten, they would likely be killed. Colonel Tarleton had a reputation for not taking many prisoners.

General Morgan's approach was totally against usual battle planning ideas, but he reasoned that with the river to their backs, every one of his men would know that they had no choice but to win. He then put together a daring but also promising battle plan, and was careful to tell his soldiers "exactly what he expected of them."[109]

His men fought hard and won a major victory.[109] The victory was partly because of General Morgan's brilliant plan and the clear instructions, but also because of his unshakeable expectation of success, which was conveyed to his men in a powerful and emotional way.

It is much the same in helping patients and their families recover from bipolar disorder. This is a major, life-threatening disorder, which many consider complex and overwhelming. Bipolar disorder leads to suicide in 10% to 15% of patients.

Many, many more bipolar patients than that, however, lose years or decades of their lives due to inability to function in their everyday lives. I therefore point out to the patient and family, "It's your life, and you have this serious disorder which is destroying you. We simply have no choice but to control the disorder so you can get back to feeling right and being able to function."

When I then point out that it will be necessary for them to become very knowledgeable about the disorder so as to improve the odds of our success, they are all ears; and the lessons I teach them during our sessions are the exact same lessons I've put in this book.

CALM SEAS

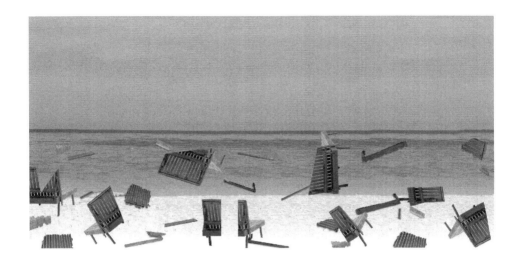

Chapter 15

Explaining and Breaking Down Hopelessness

(Or...Amazing "Blast Everything That Moves!"
Medicine Combinations, The High-Speed Spin
Cycle,
and The Dazed, Walking Zombie Half-Death)

Case 15.1

I recently saw a new patient in her 30s for an initial evaluation, Mrs. J, and that evaluation and a telephone contact shortly thereafter told me that I would need to spend a little more time than usual actively dismantling the hopelessness that Mrs. J was bringing with her to the start of her treatment with me.

She had reported a treatment many years earlier with a primary doctor just recently out of training, and when the young primary doctor heard that my patient suffered with bipolar disorder, the doctor impulsively and tellingly blurted out, "Oh, bipolar disorder, that's one of those mental disorders that's not treatable." The young primary doctor wasn't comfortable with the mood stabilizers (not unlike many clinicians who treat bipolar disorder today) and admitted this to my patient.   Because of the doctor's discomfort with the mood stabilizers, the primary doctor then essentially said to Mrs. J, "Why don't we try the antidepressants for a while, and see how it goes?"

The patient then had a few more years of treatment after that first encounter, both with other primary doctors and with psychiatrists, none of whom ever took her off the antidepressants.

Unfortunately, by the time Mrs. J eventually arrived in my office, the most urgent question on my new patient's mind was still the question of whether bipolar disorder was treatable or not. By her behavior, tone of voice, interaction with me, and almost immediate telephone call right after our first visit, it was pretty clear that she was still convinced that her bipolar disorder could not be treated successfully.

The reason I'm writing this chapter (and this book) is that a high proportion of the patients coming to me have been in treatment for many years, have had numerous trials of different treatments, and have experienced many treatment failures.   The conclusion they draw from this is that they must have a very difficult and untreatable type of illness, and that their situation is hopeless.

On looking carefully over the specific treatments that they have received over the years, I see a very different situation.   In general the medicines and medication combinations tried over the years are at odds with the established scientific findings, and have little if any chance of helping the patient reach long-term stable recovery.[18,20,21,25,26,131,210] q   As nearly as I can tell, the prior treating clinicians had been acting in good faith, but were not aware of the above issues.

The patients usually tell me on their own, or answer my question to the same effect, that they do believe they are indeed a hopeless case.   I then explain

---

q Stable recovery is described in one recent research study as at least two months of relatively stable mood, with no major mood episodes.[18] and in another, as 6 months with no major mood episodes.[20] Obviously, in clinical practice, we are working to establish a much longer recovery.

to them that their situation isn't at all hopeless. I further explain to them that instead, unfortunately, they have spent years on medication treatments and combinations that had very little chance of success.

The main reason for this seems to be that the conceptually sound approaches well known to bipolar specialists for decades, and supported by the overwhelming majority of large, high-quality scientific studies, are no longer taught to psychiatric residents and other mental health trainees at most training programs, and have been all but forgotten.[8,9,20,92,93]

Instead, psychiatric residents and psychiatric nurse practitioner trainees at many institutions learn at the hospital bedside (and also in the outpatient clinic) how to treat the patients' condition symptom by symptom.[106] A medicine is given for this symptom, and a medicine for that symptom, etc. Before you know it, the patient's medicine list has swollen to 4 to 7 medications. Unfortunately, it all happens so quickly that it is very hard to tell which medication actually does what.

These same strategies are then continued as the ongoing treatment when the hospitalized patient is discharged from the hospital into office or clinic follow-up. These complicated medication combinations are continued further for as long as they seem adequate to keep the patient out of hospital, whether the patient ever reaches stable recovery and the ability to function well again or not. Often they do not.[20,21]

Case 15.2

Mrs. K, a woman in her late 30s, had mood symptoms since her mid-teens. Then, in her early 20s, she started having euphoric ("top of the world!") manias lasting up to 1-2 weeks each. During the manias she had marked insomnia, including bouts of not sleeping at all for 4-5 days at a time. The diagnosis of bipolar disorder was missed for 8 years, and she was eventually diagnosed with bipolar disorder when she was about 30 years old.

She was treated for 2 years around age 20 by her family doctor with Ativan/lorazepam. Thereafter she was treated most of the time by psychiatrists, including during 4 of the past 5 years. Medicines prescribed over the years included newer antipsychotics, antidepressants, benzodiazepines, and divalproex.

Mrs. K could not recall ever having been treated with a mood stabilizer all by itself. She had instead always been treated with multiple medicines, often 5 to 8 medicines at once, and sometimes with 4 new medicines started all at once, but she had never experienced a full or stable recovery. The large medicine combinations sometimes put her into a zombie-like state, against which she understandably rebelled.

Severe irritability had been a major factor in two of her psychiatric hospitalizations on the psychiatric ward of a university-affiliated teaching hospital, including her very recent 5-day stay there. Mrs. K had been on Paxil 40 mg/day, Trazodone 50 mg 3 times a day, Klonopin 1 mg twice a day, and Ambien 10 mg at bedtime for the past 2 years, with no benefit. She continued to sleep only 3 to 4 hours per night.

After the above most recent hospitalization, Mrs. K was referred to a public clinic for follow-up care. At the initial psychiatric evaluation there, she reported she felt desperate about her condition, as she wasn't eating or sleeping since leaving the hospital. She appeared moody and at times tearful, but very cooperative. She gave a clear history of distinct, euphoric ("top of the world!") manias in the past, which might predict a higher likelihood of a good response to lithium given all by itself,[4] but this had never been tried with her.

Accordingly, after a lengthy evaluation and discussion of all the above with the patient, the public clinic psychiatrist added lithium while simultaneously tapering and discontinuing all her prior medicines.

When Mrs. K was seen for a follow-up appointment 9 weeks later, she was only on lithium 600 mg at bedtime. She appeared much calmer. She reported that rather than sleeping 3 to 4 hours per night as she had before, that she was now sleeping 6 to 7 hours per night, waking up rested, and with noticeably better daytime energy. She was, by her own report, 80% better than when first seen on 4 medicines, and she felt the best she had felt in 18 years.

The above unnecessary 18-year delay in Mrs. K getting relief for a severe but very treatable illness is commonplace. Unfortunately, no one seems to teach the trainees at teaching institutions which medications have actually been shown by scientific study to be effective in bipolar disorder over the long term, and which ones have not, and therefore how to remodel the complex medication combinations into simpler combinations that might actually help the patient improve further after hospital discharge.[20,21,41,92,93,210]

Now bear in mind that hospital doctors and teaching faculty are very intelligent, extremely hard working clinicians. The problem comes about in part because the hospital team has to treat an unbelievable number of extremely ill, often suicidal, occasionally homicidal patients extremely fast, often in only 2-5 hospital days, and discharge these relatively unstable patients in improved and more stable condition within these extremely short time frames, which are often faster than many of the medications really have time to be effective.

In the hospital (and also if the patient is instead being seen first in the outpatient office), clinicians often start the patient with an antidepressant, because almost every bipolar patient arrives with suicide thoughts and urges, and/or complains in some way about feeling depressed[69,94,131] (See also Chapters 5 and 16). These sometimes superficial descriptions are then sometimes taken fairly quickly, and without asking a lot more specific questions, to mean a full, pure bipolar depressive episode, which they often do not.

As noted in Chapter 3, and elsewhere, this is the beginning of building a polarity-based medicine regimen with antidepressants paired with antipsychotics (usually the atypical antipsychotics) used as anti-manic coverage. It is thereby felt that one has covered both "poles" (up and down) of the "bi-polar" disorder.[24,106] Unfortunately, such regimens employing antidepressants are not usually effective in long-term treatment.[10,12,13,16,18,19,20,21,25,26,28,29,38,39,40,41,210]

Just recently, some clinicians have started treating bipolar patients with an antidepressant plus Lamictal (lamotrigine) instead, which unfortunately is perhaps even less reasonable, as lamotrigine is only a weak antimanic or ceiling, thus leaving the patient even more vulnerable to breakout to the upside, into manic or mixed worsening, as also described in Chapter 8, and in Case 15.3 below.

Case 15.3

Ms. M was already in office treatment with a psychiatrist for well-established bipolar I disorder. Almost all of her mood episodes had been manias. These had responded very well to lithium. She had been doing extremely well, and continued to work full time while on lithium as her only medication for several months prior to this episode.

The new episode came in the context of dramatically increased life pressures. Ms. M then had a serious breakdown including experiencing some brief psychotic features (some loss of touch with reality). She was therefore hospitalized for a few days at a university-affiliated teaching hospital.

The hospital team continued the lithium, and added an SSRI antidepressant for the patient's tendency to obsess, which they felt might be an even more important disorder than her bipolar disorder. The next night, however, Ms. M did not sleep, suggesting the antidepressant was triggering or worsening a manic or mixed episode. The team therefore stopped the antidepressant. They also stopped her lithium (a powerful anti-manic), and replaced it with lamotrigine (Lamictal, a weak anti-manic).

Forty-eight hours after discharge from hospital, the office psychiatrist received a call from Ms. M that she was experiencing worsening insomnia and other manic symptoms. The office psychiatrist therefore added the lithium back into her regimen, and continued the lamotrigine, as lamotrigine is a mood stabilizer, and not known to worsen manic episodes. The manic symptoms, as well as the psychotic features, resolved rapidly over the next few days in response to adding the lithium back in.

The tendency to obsess was a long-standing part of Ms. M's personality, and might be expected to respond more successfully to psychotherapy (talk therapy) after first achieving several more weeks of mood stability while back on the lithium.

For successful treatment of the above and other cases, please refer to Chapter 12 on hierarchic diagnosis, to review the rank order of disorders by urgency. Until the more urgent disorders are well controlled, attempts to treat less urgent disorders, such as obsessing, are likely to fail. This is in part because the more urgent disorders may mimic or worsen the less urgent disorders. In this case, the particular treatment of the obsessions (SSRI antidepressant medicine) is also known to have the potential to worsen the more urgent condition, the bipolar disorder.

We return now to the routine modern construction of hospital medicine combinations (and often also of outpatient office or clinic medicine combinations): After the first 2 medicines (antidepressant and antipsychotic[r]) are started, one then adds in hospital, during the usual brief 2-5 day hospital stay, a number of other medicines. These are intended to treat whatever the patient might report from the Chinese menu of symptoms and symptom complexes.

Many patients are therefore given trazodone or Remeron (mirtazapine) for insomnia (antidepressants known to occasionally precipitate manic or mixed episodes, or worsening of cycling), or Ambien (zolpidem), or another conventional "sleeper" such as Restoril (temazepam).

They're then often given another medicine for their anxiety, such as a benzodiazepine, or Buspar (buspirone) or Neurontin (gabapentin), or Vistaril (hydroxyzine).[s]

The patient might then also need an anti-restlessness medication to combat the restlessness from the antipsychotic, an anti-panic medication, a medicine for poor concentration, etc., etc. Getting to a medicine combination of 4 to 7 medications becomes a piece of cake.

Case 15.4

A 28 year old man with manic episodes since age 16 was eventually diagnosed with bipolar disorder at age 22, and also suffered with alcoholism. At discharge from his most recent psychiatric hospitalization for bipolar disorder, his regimen consisted of Lexapro (antidepressant), Seroquel (antipsychotic), Abilify (antipsychotic), Buspar (anti-anxiety), Neurontin (anti-anxiety), Vistaril (anti-anxiety), and Naltrexone (anti-alcohol cravings). Note that this regimen had 7 psychiatric medicines, including an antidepressant, but no traditional mood stabilizers, as is commonly the case with polarity-based regimens (see Chapter 3).

When seen for outpatient follow-up by a different doctor, he reported

---

r or occasionally antidepressant and lamotrigine

s It is only rarely noted that disruptive insomnia and anxiety are manic or mixed symptoms (symptoms of over-activation, as described in Chapters 16 and 17) and might therefore be treated more simply with an adjusted dose of one or even two mood stabilizers, or a mood stabilizer and an atypical antipsychotic (Chapters 8 and 9). These need to be given in the absence of antidepressants, as antidepressants have been linked to worse cycling,[4,19,27] manias,[37,39] mixed states,[12,13,25,26,68] depressions,[12,25,26] and suicidal behaviors.[38,59]

moderate-to-severe mixed bipolar symptoms, with somewhat more severe manic symptoms (as compared to the severity of his depressive symptoms at that point in time). This would be described as a manic mixed episode (MMX, as described in Chapter 5). If continued, the antidepressant would be likely to make his overall condition worse.[12,13,25,26,68]

The anxiety, which required 3 different medicines, might have been more effectively treated by very slow taper of the antidepressant (Chapters 10 and 13) and the addition of 1 or more mood stabilizers. One could thereby treat the underlying illness rather than the surface symptoms.

Time is only rarely taken in modern-day practice to ask the lifetime history of all mood episodes, and to be sure of having the correct primary diagnosis first, after which the medicine regimen can be built out in an evidence-based manner as needed to address the core primary illness. When one does this properly, many of the other symptoms, such as insomnia, anxiety, problems concentrating, and feeling down, vanish rapidly.

Instead there is nowadays the assumption that there is a suitable medication for any symptom the patient may describe, regardless of the primary diagnosis. It's almost as if there is more focus on individual symptoms than there is on the more likely idea that most of the patient's symptoms may be expressions of the core primary illness.

That is, "A drug for every symptom" rather than "Let's evaluate very carefully to be sure we've got the right primary disorder, which we'll then treat according to sound evidence-based principles for that disorder."[t]

This complex polypharmacy (many medicines) may, of course, seem to work in the short term to get the patient out of the hospital. For one thing, the patient learns at some point that voicing any symptoms at all might result in their getting more medicines and staying in hospital longer, and they usually just want to get out.

The problem is that these regimens, which may seem somewhat effective in hospital, may be very sedating, and the side effects of all these medicines may make it difficult for the patient to function in real life outside the hospital. The hospital medicines, however, are rarely if ever readjusted, even if they don't

---

t The correct primary diagnosis is most likely to be arrived at by a process that includes the idea of top-down or "hierarchic" diagnosis (diagnosis rank ordered by urgency and severity), which is discussed in Chapter 12.

succeed in helping the patient reach stable recovery during outpatient treatment.

In the long-term treatment of patients, it is extremely important to reach stable recovery (as described above) and maintain patients in stable recovery for many months, and preferably for years, so that they can start rebuilding their lives.

The medicines most likely to help patients get to stable recovery are the inexpensive but extremely effective mood stabilizers. Unfortunately, these are avoided nowadays like the plague, as they are "old medicines" (not hip or trendy). They are also thought (probably incorrectly) to be "toxic," or dangerous, by many fully-trained and even experienced clinicians. This belief suggests that these clinicians were possibly never trained in how to manage these medicines safely.

There are certainly potential hazards with the mood stabilizers, and safe management requires a bit more oversight and monitoring. It is not rocket science, however, and it can be taught easily. Some of the safety concerns and monitoring issues have already been described in Chapter 9. Patients and family can also be taught how to assist with the monitoring.

The newer and more popular medications have been more actively marketed by the pharmaceutical companies, and seem easier to manage in the beginning. The newer medications, however, may actually be more hazardous in the ongoing maintenance phase, which stretches on for years, as opposed to the acute treatment phase, which lasts only days to weeks.

Very interestingly, when these 'ancient' mood stabilizers (now some 30 to 40 years old) are skillfully applied (with or without the newer antipsychotics, and with or without the newer mood stabilizer lamotrigine/Lamictal, but without the antidepressants), they provide nice bedtime sedation and anxiety reduction that often make some of the other medications unnecessary. They thus permit building smaller,[41] better tolerated, and more effective medicine combinations for the long run.[20,21,131,143,210] The patient can be treated and stabilized and rehabilitated successfully without becoming a "zombie."

When I keep emphasizing "the long run," please bear in mind that bipolar disorder is a lifelong disorder. It seems to me to be high time that we taught our trainees not just that which is convenient, rapid, 'newer and therefore better,' and seemingly effective in the short run, but also that which has been scientifically demonstrated to be most effective in the long run.

After hospitalization or other acute treatment, adjustments often need to be made, focused on the goal of long-term stable recovery.[143,190,210] The medicines started in hospital are not necessarily sacred; they are just what it took to quiet the acute episode. The medicine combinations used for long-term maintenance are actually more important to the prospect of long-term success.

Consider the results of a 2-year study of 1,656 bipolar I patients entering maintenance treatment for an acute manic/mixed episode: "Prescription of typical antipsychotics and antidepressants at the first visit of the long-term treatment phase (12 weeks) were independent predictors of lower remission and recovery rates."[210] That is, if patients entering long-term treatment were prescribed either antidepressants or older antipsychotics, they had less complete clearing of symptoms, and lower rates of returning to full functioning.

Unfortunately, in the modern scenario, the treatment begun during the acute episode is often continued so long as it manages to keep the patient quiet enough to stay out of the hospital most of the time. It's therefore not surprising that when the patients don't reach a stable recovery,[18,20] that the patients would conclude that their nonproductive and emotionally painful condition must be the result of a hopeless disorder.

Some of the patients coming to see me have even had the boldness to ask their prior doctors whether this is as good as it gets, i.e., a sort of agitated, irritable, unstable, over-sedated, walking zombie half-death with ongoing uncontrolled mood cycling and mood episodes. Their prior doctors, mostly psychiatrists, have reportedly almost always told them that yes, this is as good as it gets, that this is as good as anyone could reasonably expect with bipolar disorder.

These patients haven't been taught the audacity to conclude instead that their treatments might be ineffective and disconnected from the scientific evidence, or sometimes even counterproductive. That is exactly what I have to teach them in an attempt to jostle them out of their hopelessness, because after a few years of treatment with the above approaches, their hopelessness is pretty deeply entrenched, and it takes quite a wallop to get them out of it.

For better or worse, I am no longer willing to offer justifications for the questionable medicine combinations on which my incoming new patients with bipolar disorder arrive at my office.[u] To do so would seem to be saying to the patients that their prior treatment was reasonable and consistent with the scientific evidence, which, unfortunately, it often is not. It would be the same as saying, "Yes dear, you really are a hopeless case," which, with the bipolar patients coming to me over the past few years, would be nonsense. None of their conditions is hopeless, so long as their treatment is carefully reevaluated, and they are willing to try a different approach.

It is my hope that the overall approach to the diagnosis and treatment of bipolar disorder will be reevaluated, so that this sort of needless tragedy happens much less often going forward.

The explanation above seems to reassure the patients a bit; however, given that I've just told them that they're not a hopeless case, and that their disorder is treatable, they continue to harbor some lingering suspicions that I might have just arrived from Mars. My clinical descriptions to them usually line up so tightly with their own experience, however, that they pull themselves back together a bit and try to give the approach I'm describing the benefit of the doubt long enough to return for a second session, and perhaps even try what I recommend.

---

u Just a brief look at these medication combinations and review of the patient's complete lifetime history of mood episodes is often enough to predict with high likelihood that these combinations would have very little chance of helping the patient to reach stable recovery.

CALM SEAS

Section D:

Confusing Common Terms,

and New Faces of Mania

CALM SEAS

Chapter 16

DEPRESSION and ANXIETY, *The Urgent Need for a New Vocabulary...*

OR... Time to Start Looking at **ACTIVATION** Instead.

Depression and anxiety are probably the two most common terms used today by patients, families, and even clinicians, to describe mood states in bipolar patients. Unfortunately, the way they're used now, these descriptions have become useless or outright misleading. This chapter offers a different, more useful way of viewing bipolar mood states.

Please consider the following definitions:

Depression, noun.

1. Any unpleasant, unwanted, painful, sad, or less than ideal feeling(s), under any conditions or circumstances whatsoever, for whatever reason, at any time or place, or for any duration, regardless of anything else.

2. In the everyday practice of clinical psychiatry, a full major depressive episode.[24]

That is, the description in #1 above is generally not carefully questioned in adequate detail, but instead is fairly rapidly assumed to be a full major depressive episode, (at least 2 weeks of serious and almost incapacitating depression with very specific depressive symptoms,[24] see Appendix). This assumption then provides the seeming justification for lurching ahead with a prescription for antidepressant medication treatment.

Anxiety, noun.

1. Any other bad feeling not described as depression, especially if one feels over-activated in any way, i.e., "wound up" or agitated.

As nearly as I can tell from my everyday observation of clinical office practice, the above descriptions encompass almost the entire state of symptom description in modern psychiatric outpatient practice today. We hear about and discuss only two feeling states, depression and anxiety. In Chapter 5, about mixed episodes, I pointed out that almost every session with almost every bipolar patient starts with the initial complaint being something along the lines of, "Doctor, I'm feeling depressed." For better or worse, the same could be said for almost every patient I see who suffers any other disorder. For a variety of reasons, we have progressed to the point where "I'm feeling depressed" essentially now means "I'm feeling bad in some way," or "I'm feeling less than completely well" in any way whatsoever.

A limited and incomplete listing of a few of the things patients describe as "depression," but which turns out to be something else on further questioning and listening follows:

Regular, expectable, and appropriate sadness, grief, or bereavement.

Arguments with the husband/wife/partner, marital or relationship tension.

Financial pressures or reverses, poverty, hunger.

Work pressures, difficult boss, difficult co-workers, hostile work environment.

Problems with children, child-rearing, disagreement with spouse over how to raise children, children with academic or behavioral problems, children forcibly removed from the home or needing short-term or long-term placement away from the family.

Emotional effects of illness in patient, spouse, or children.

Overwhelming demands of working, often full time, as well as raising children and maintaining the household, especially if one is a single parent.

Alcohol or drug abuse in the patient, spouse, children, or other relatives.

Needing to care for an aging parent or parents, and finding oneself overwhelmed doing so.

Chronic pain, chronic fatigue, or sleep apnea.

Direct effects of many medical, surgical, or neurological illnesses, chronic or acute.

Side effects of psychotropic or other medications, including sedation, emotional blunting, interference with energy and/or motivation, etc.

Current abusive relationship and/or residual trauma from childhood abuse.

Ran out of medications, took medications improperly, took someone else's medications.

Inability to function due to manic or mixed state.

Understandable discouragement and just feeling drained in the lifelong process of dealing with chronic or recurrent bipolar disorder, sometimes because the treatment is too costly in time, money, and effort, especially if the treatment is ineffective.

Sometimes these situations are accompanied by a clear depressive illness, but much more often they are not. In such situations it is wise not to try to treat an episode of bipolar depressive illness where none exists, as this often makes the condition worse and less treatable.

As just another example of how completely this way of viewing every emotional disruption or condition as depression or anxiety has seeped into our psychiatric culture, there is a clinic in our area that specializes in diagnostic screening of new patients. As part of their standard evaluation, they administer two proven screening instruments, one for depression and the other for anxiety. Now there are quite a few good screening instruments for the full range of psychiatric illnesses, including bipolar disorder, schizophrenia, and others,[212] but the only ones administered are for depression and anxiety.

How did we get here?

In the 1980s depression was not diagnosed nearly as often as it perhaps should have been. The medication treatments for depression available at that time were associated with bothersome side effects and were somewhat hazardous, and potentially lethal in overdose. The treatment of depression was therefore often delegated to the medical specialists in mental disorders, the psychiatrists. Unfortunately, then, as now, there weren't enough psychiatrists to go around.

As a result of depression not being diagnosed enough and patients not having enough treatment avenues, there was a major public awareness campaign launched in 1993 as a joint venture of the United States Department of Health and Human Services,[160] together with healthcare professionals, academic institutions, and the pharmaceutical industry. This campaign aimed to alert patients, families, and clinicians how they could spot depression more readily. There was also the hope and intention that family doctors and other primary health care doctors might identify and treat more of the depressed patients.

The movement toward more identification and treatment of depression had actually begun in late 1987 and in 1988, when Prozac (fluoxetine) burst on the scene. The arrival of Prozac changed everything.[117] Prozac was the first in the hugely successful SSRI (selective serotonin reuptake inhibitor) class of antidepressants. Wellbutrin (bupropion, not an SSRI) arrived at about the same time, but wasn't quite such an instant success. Zoloft was approved in 1992, and Paxil in 1994, and these two were also instant successes for the pharmaceutical companies who developed and marketed them.

These new agents revolutionized the treatment of depression, just as society was being alerted to how common it is. The new antidepressants were overall a good deal safer than the prior antidepressants (primarily the tricyclic antidepressants), and easier to administer and monitor. One could prescribe a full therapeutic dose immediately at the start of treatment with some, or within 1 week with the others.

This was much easier than with the earlier medications, which required a gradual build-up to full treatment doses over several days to a few weeks. High enough doses of the earlier medicines were often never reached in clinical practice. As a result, the psychiatric consultants to the makers of Prozac lobbied the company hard not to even offer a dose lower than a full therapeutic dose, that is, one 20 mg capsule taken once daily.

With more easily tolerated medicines given at full doses, patients, families, clinicians, and even society at large, all saw that depression had become much more treatable than before, sometimes with dramatically better results,[117] and all the above groups very understandably became enchanted with these new SSRIs and Wellbutrin. Treatment was therefore started in the primary care doctors' offices more, and primary care doctors became much more confident diagnosing and treating depression themselves, just as the national awareness campaign had hoped. Doctors also began to see that the SSRI antidepressants could be used to treat many more conditions than just depression.[117]

It should be noted, however, that there was never any such large-scale nationwide campaign to educate primary doctors and other healthcare providers about the diagnosis and treatment of bipolar disorder.[v]

If a patient then failed a trial of an antidepressant because of developing fairly prominent manic symptoms or even a full manic or mixed episode, it was likely instead to be viewed simply as an antidepressant treatment failure. It would generally be assumed that the antidepressant simply wasn't the best one for this particular patient. Most often, then, if increasing the dose of the original antidepressant hadn't helped, this situation would lead to the doctor switching the patient to a different antidepressant, rather than re-evaluating whether or not the initial depression diagnosis was accurate.

The fates of anxiety took some slightly different turns, only to end up in the same neighborhood. Even in the 1980s, we had highly effective medications for anxiety, the benzodiazepines (BZs), and these are still prescribed today. These were much safer than the extremely risky and addictive barbiturates they

---

v As an example of how, even today, depression and anxiety continue to be viewed as common and important, and bipolar disorder continues to be treated as if uncommon and/or less important, the 2013 Annual Meeting of the American Psychiatric Association offered numerous official courses whose descriptions mentioned depression and/or anxiety as major topics for discussion, but not a single course devoted primarily to bipolar disorder.[168]

replaced, but even the BZs still had moderate addictive risk, which limited their use somewhat in the 1980s, and limits their use even more today.

A funny thing happened along the way, though. Even as the SSRI antidepressants were getting a lock on the treatment of depression, it was also being discovered that they were highly effective for most anxiety disorders,[117] and they started pushing aside the BZs as the treatment of choice for most anxiety. The primary care doctors and others, who had already become extremely comfortable with using the SSRIs for depression treatment, were now even more enthusiastic about them, as they also seemed to treat anxiety successfully. At the same time, these doctors were having ongoing misgivings about the use of the BZs for anxiety.

In addition to the potential the BZs had to trigger or worsen possible addictions in those for whom they were prescribed, the BZs also had the potential to be "diverted" (misdirected) to sale on the street, where they brought very good prices from addicts or dealers. If a doctor prescribed a lot of them, this might bring the unwanted negative attention of colleagues, pharmacists, and even the state medical board, which in extreme cases might suspend or revoke one's license to practice. Thus there was and is a huge incentive to switch patients from the BZs to the SSRIs.

Some of these patients, however, have been on medium to high doses of BZs for up to 20 years or more, and now are in their 50s or 60s or even older. Some are medically frail.

Such a changeover from the BZs to the SSRIs (or SNRIs) is not at all easy under such circumstances. In my opinion, many clinicians underestimate how difficult it will be to transition from the BZs to the SSRIs, and they underestimate by a significant amount how long it would take to be successful, if this is even possible with a long-term patient such as this. There is also no guarantee that a given patient who responds successfully to the BZs will also respond well to the SSRIs.

Unfortunately, under the above pressures, some primary care clinicians simply try to dump the problem by refusing to continue the BZs that they or their practice group or colleagues may have prescribed for years, and telling the patient they'll have to get them from a psychiatrist.

In any event, the interesting outcome is that now a huge proportion of patients with both depression and anxiety disorders are treated with SSRIs, or the newer version with overall similar properties, the SNRIs (serotonin and norepinephrine reuptake inhibitors). So in a very real way, the above diagnostic clinic using proven screening instruments only for depression and anxiety, might be considered to be screening for people likely to respond well to the SSRIs and the SNRIs. What the patients with other disorders are to do is apparently not quite as clear.

All these changes over the past 25 years have also played out in our society's perception of mental and emotional disorders. The feeling is now that the disorders that regular people get are depression and anxiety, the disorders that respond to SSRIs, SNRIs, and other antidepressants.

On the other hand, there is the perception that if you get some condition other than depression or anxiety, you must be "crazy." Accordingly, the emotions that people expect to experience are also perceived as depression and/or anxiety, and so these have become what almost all patients tell their doctors.

Even the briefest mention of "depression" is often taken to mean that the patient must be suffering a full major depressive episode, and thus a prescription for a newer antidepressant is often written immediately by the increasingly busy and overwhelmed practitioner, as these medicines are highly likely to be helpful, right?

In one way this is a good thing for some folks, as if makes it easier for them to enter treatment, if this is what they suffer. In another way, however, it's kind of weird, as if depression and anxiety have completely replaced our prior knowledge and description and discussion of all other human feeling states.

So is there a helpful way we can move forward past these limitations?

(As a truth in advertising moment, I should remind you that I am a bipolar specialist. I am also aware of the helpful warning, "If the tool you have is a hammer, every problem starts to look like a nail;" but please read on.)

The people left out by the total focus on depression and anxiety in our thinking include, among others, the patients with bipolar disorder, specifically those with bipolar I disorder (obvious symptoms and severe impact) and bipolar II disorder (moderate symptoms with moderate impact of the episodes,[24] but sometimes every bit as rocky a long-term clinical course as bipolar I). (See Glossary, and also Appendix for formal diagnostic descriptions.) The situation isn't as clear for those with bipolar disorder NOS (not otherwise specified, which generally has less obvious symptoms and less severe impact).[24,184,185]

It has, however, been my repeated experience, now hundreds of times, that, when the bipolar disorder is detected or labeled at all, many clinicians diagnose bipolar disorder at 1 or 2 notches lower on the severity scale than the patient's actual clinical course deserves. That is, they often diagnose the patient as having bipolar disorder NOS when the patient actually suffers the more severe bipolar I or II disorder. Many, many other times they diagnose the patient as having bipolar II disorder, when the patient actually has bipolar I disorder.

Occasionally this is just diagnosing overly cautiously due to being in a rush to see a lot of patients very fast. At other times it may involve the clinician trying to protect the patient from the significant perceived stigma (and discrimination by insurance companies and others) of having a more serious condition.

While I respect the wish to try to protect the patient from stigma and discrimination, it is my opinion that it is more important to apply the correct diagnosis. This improves the odds of getting the patient on the correct path to a successful treatment approach and a good outcome. Having a more "politically correct" diagnosis is little comfort, in my opinion, if you're unable to function due to bipolar disorder still running wild and destroying your life.

The result of the above tendency to "softer diagnosis" is that the risks of unsuccessful treatment and inability to reach stable recovery being discussed here with regard to bipolar I and II disorders may actually apply to many who are currently diagnosed as having bipolar disorder NOS.[24]

Please see the DSM-IV-TR descriptions of the symptoms required to diagnose the above disorders[24] in Appendix 1.

As mentioned in previous chapters, the problem here is that SSRIs, SNRIs, and other antidepressants do not help in the vast majority of bipolar I and bipolar II patients, and they may more often be associated with things getting worse.

Unfortunately, as noted above, we haven't yet put forth even a fraction of the time and effort educating clinicians about bipolar disorder that we have about depression, and therefore, even when things go badly because the patient has bipolar disorder rather than major depressive disorder, this may not be recognized as the problem.

Bipolar patients in study after study routinely have serious bipolar symptoms for 5 to 16 years before receiving the correct diagnosis of their bipolar disorder,[58,63-66, 69,156,201,202] and therefore they may also go 5 to 16 years with treatments more likely to be associated with worsening of their condition rather than improvement.

I have a suggestion that may help both with the extreme limiting of our language to only two words to describe all human emotions, as well as the risk of bipolar patients remaining undetected, and thereby receiving unhelpful treatment.[182,200]

It is the introduction of the dimension of **ACTIVATION**,[79,206] which includes over-activation, normal activation, and under-activation. This is, of course, a sneaky way of introducing bipolar concepts into the depression-only world and vocabulary of the 1990s, 2000s, and 2010s.

In an important recent study,[206] activation "proved to be the most potent discriminator of those with unipolar versus bipolar diagnoses." Translation: Higher levels of activation were the most effective marker to sort out bipolar patients from patients with major depressive disorder. It is interesting to consider which DSM-IV-TR[24] symptoms distinguish bipolar disorder from major depressive disorder. It turns out that these are manic symptoms. It would follow then that high levels of activation, or over-activation, would indicate a high likelihood of manic symptoms, which are present in manic or mixed episodes.

Over-activation may involve any wound-up, revved-up, over-energized state. This may include agitation, irritability, rage, euphoria, grandiosity, high anxiety, high energy, high sex drive or excessive sexual activity, talking way too much, doing too much and too many different things, acting on impulse, engaging in high-risk behaviors, becoming very distracted, and having racing thoughts or crowded thoughts or way too many thoughts all at once. It may also involve having trouble sleeping, often because of the high energy and because the racing mind and body won't let the patient rest. If this condition goes on untreated or unsuccessfully treated for long periods of time, it may in some cases lead to more dangerous behaviors, alcohol or drug abuse, loss of contact with reality, confusion, dehydration, or physical exhaustion and collapse.

In my experience (in contrast to the official description in DSM-IV-TR[24] that the insomnia involves decreased need for sleep), the patient often wants more sleep, is well aware that he or she needs more sleep, tries repeatedly to get more sleep, but just simply can't quiet the racing mind and body.

Some observers have described decreased sleep, even in patients with well-established bipolar I or bipolar II disorder, as "depressive insomnia"[121,122] if the patient can't sleep but does need sleep. This seems very unreasonable to me because of the following.

Insomnia often begins in childhood, and often as the very first symptom of bipolar disorder.[56,203] As a result, by the time the patients come to see me in their 20s, 30s, 40s, or 50s, they are usually well into the late course of bipolar disorder (Chapters 4 and 5). A significant proportion of them have rapidly shifting mixed states with insomnia, and a high proportion of them have been severely sleep deprived for years or even decades.

They're feeling racy, anxious, edgy, and irritable, but **exhausted**, and in urgent need of better sleep, and they're often well aware they need more sleep. They just simply can't wind down. In such situations, restoring normal sleep, and a normal sleep-wake cycle, becomes the first treatment priority (Chapter 6).

Now note that these patients are not having trouble sleeping due to under-activation; they're having trouble sleeping due to **over-activation**, almost always accompanied by some other indicators of over-activation, such as racing thoughts, distractibility, irritability, impulsivity, etc.[206]

Therefore, in my opinion and experience, in a patient with well-established bipolar I or II disorder, if the patient can't sleep despite good effort and clear intention to do so, and is sleeping less than 6 hours per night, or substantially less than their usual amount of sleep when well, then this is a manic component of a manic or mixed state (see Duffy's Rule in Chapter 6).

To try to require the sleep to be un-needed to be considered manic or mixed-episode insomnia is just simply unreasonable under these circumstances, and may be quite misleading.[122] This may be one of the reasons, for example, for the substantial underdiagnosis of manic and mixed states as part of treatment as usual.[63-65,69,79,94,140]

Under-activation is present when one has no energy, no interest, takes no pleasure in anything, feels no motivation, loses social interest in loved ones and people in general, loses sexual interest and drive, often sleeps too much,[146] and often doesn't have enough energy or interest to do anything else. It may seem as if they're spray-painted on the couch or bed, and just barely alive. They often sleep too much or even stay in bed awake in an attempt to try to escape from the horrible feeling state they're experiencing. They can lose interest to the degree where they see no point in living at all. Whereas the over-activated person is often flooded with thoughts, the under-activated patient doesn't have enough energy to have much constructive mental activity at all, and what little there is has a very negative tinge. It's as if their whole body and mind are shut down, and they just wish everybody and everything would go away and leave them alone.

You will have noticed that what I have described as under-activation has a lot of the features we might think of when we're thinking of moderate or severe depression. On the other hand, just think over for a moment how much is contained in the idea of over-activation, as described in the paragraphs above. Think of how little of this over-activation is covered by the term of "anxiety," as also shown in figure 16.1.

Figure 16.1

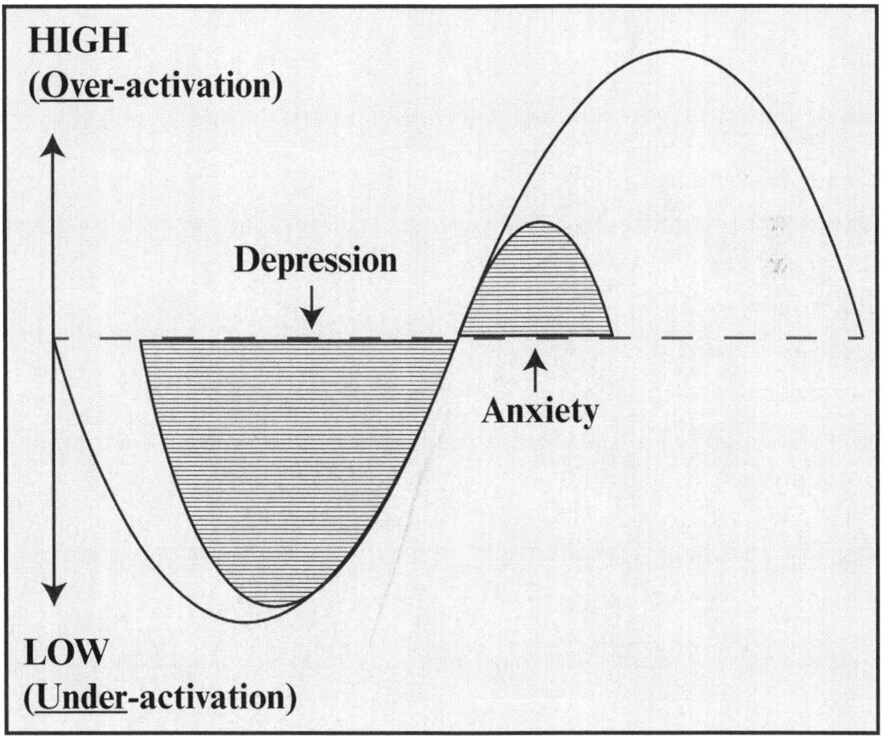

HIGH
(Over-activation)

Depression

Anxiety

LOW
(Under-activation)

This is the part that our current vocabulary and our current way of thinking is missing, and much of the over-activation that isn't covered by the term of anxiety should tip us off to the possibility of previously unsuspected manic or mixed episode, thereby indicating a bipolar disorder. In those with known bipolar disorder, reported high anxiety, just as reported severe insomnia, should immediately have us thinking of, and listening and looking for mania or mixed state.

Let me offer as just one example of over-activation that isn't fully covered by anxiety, Hilary's story, which she kindly offered to share with you (Case 16.1):

Case 16.1

"While in the hospital after my suicide, the nurses and my psychiatrist were very impressed with my energy, conversation in groups, and my involvement with other patients. I literally knew every patient in the ward and their disorder in two days – I was manic. I was released from the hospital because I was doing 'so well.'

My antidepressant drugs had been increased, which may have led to my 'speedy' recovery – no pun intended. I was flitting around there like an idiot. Now that I think back on it, it was just hilarious."

Note that at the time, neither the doctor, nor the patient, nor the nursing staff identified her racy behavior as anything other than a desirable recovery from depression. This occurred despite her staying up until 3 a.m., and talking at length with the only other patient up at that hour, who was also suffering, as you might have guessed, a manic episode.

This is a striking example of a patient with a mood and energy state not adequately described as depression or anxiety, but instead as an entirely different form of over-activation, requiring an entirely different diagnostic and treatment approach.

Chapter 17

Severe Anxiety: A Possible Third Type of Mania?

When considering the possibility of mania, most clinicians and patients tend to think of euphoric, bubbly, "top of the world" mania. Yet cranky, irritable, explosive mania is probably a good deal more common. But what if there were yet even a third presentation of mania, one which had until now been described infrequently, if at all? Consider the following cases:

Case 17.1: This involves a note to a public clinic psychiatrist from the patient's case manager (a front-line clinician who works with patients on basic issues such as money, jobs, and housing):

The case manager reported she had moved the patient's appointment with the psychiatrist earlier due to the patient experiencing "severe anxiety." When the patient tried to sleep he experienced heart racing, hot and cold rushes, inability to stop thinking, and feeling as if his head was a gerbil on a gerbil wheel. He had trouble falling asleep, trouble staying asleep, and was only getting about 4 to 6 hours of sleep per night. He was also having some mild hallucinations.

The case manager and the patient were wondering why the psychiatrist was suspecting bipolar disorder. They were also requesting a nighttime medication that would control the anxiety so that he could sleep better.

Now looking at this from the point of view of activation discussed in the last chapter, would you say this patient was over-activated or under-activated?

Note that the case manager was thinking that the patient probably needed a sleep medicine, such as possibly Ambien (zolpidem), and possibly an anxiety medicine, such as Ativan (lorazepam) or Klonopin (clonazepam). Note how the psychiatrist finds a different way to address the insomnia and anxiety.

Given the prominent anxiety, racing thoughts, trouble falling asleep and staying asleep, significant overall insomnia with only 4 to 6 hours per night of sleep, and some hallucinations, the psychiatrist noted a pattern of considerable over-activation.[44] By asking a few more questions and applying standard DSM-IV-TR criteria[24], he diagnosed bipolar I mania[24] and discussed this with the patient, and also with the case manager. Because of the diagnosis of bipolar I mania, the psychiatrist started the patient on the mood stabilizer Depakote (divalproex), and reduced the patient's antidepressant Prozac (fluoxetine), with the plan to stop the Prozac at one of the next follow-up visits.

When the patient saw the psychiatrist again 7 weeks later, the patient was on Depakote 500 mg in the morning and 1000 mg at bedtime. Rather than the gradual reductions the doctor had recommended, the patient had taken himself off the Prozac altogether, with no major problem.

The patient was now sleeping much more soundly, 6 to 8 hours per night, and waking up more rested. He was noticeably calmer and more optimistic. He could see that he was likely to improve even further, as previously described in Chapter 6.

The improvement in sleep was significant, but not yet fully back to normal. The patient was markedly calmer, but still somewhat over-activated. Therefore, the psychiatrist increased the Depakote further from 1500 mg/day to 2000 mg/day, and ordered a Depakote level and lab studies for 1 week later. The lab results would help guide further adjustments in Depakote if these were needed to control the patient's manic episode more completely.

In summary, rather than adding a sleep medicine and an anti-anxiety medicine, the psychiatrist added a mood stabilizer and increased it fairly rapidly to a dose likely to be effective in controlling the mania, and thereby also the associated anxiety. The antidepressant was reduced, and then stopped. The patient improved markedly, and there was no need for sleep medicine or anti-anxiety medicine.

Case 17.2: Mrs. N, a patient in her late 30s with a well-established diagnosis of bipolar disorder called the answering service on the weekend reporting, "Severe anxiety and depression. Meds are not helping."

She had recently been started in the office on an atypical antipsychotic (AAP, anti-manic medicine, see Glossary). After being on the AAP a few days, it appeared to have led to two trips to the ER with migraine, so the doctor covering for me at that time had taken her off the atypical AAP.

She then apparently retried the AAP on her own and experienced panic attacks, despite already being on a low dose of the anti-anxiety medication Ativan (lorazepam). She was having substantial difficulty functioning as a mother with her young children. She had chronic and significant but essentially unchanged life pressures.

Now to my way of thinking, severe anxiety is a form of over-activation,[44,206] as contrasted for instance with the most pronounced state of under-activation, sleep, during which most people aren't experiencing anxiety.

Over-activation in my view suggests mania,[44,206] so I asked how many hours she was sleeping per night, and she said 4 to 6 hours per night. She would then wake up with anxiety and nausea. When asked, she reported she also had racing thoughts, distractibility, impulsivity, and irritability. She did, of course, report feeling bad with all the above, but there was no spontaneous description of, nor tone of, depression, hopelessness, etc.

In summary, she had an apparent manic episode, not controlled by the AAP, with manifestations including insomnia and disruptive anxiety. In asking about prior medications tried (and keeping in mind her recurrence of migraine), the patient acknowledged that she had previously been on the mood stabilizer and anti-migraine medication Depakote (divalproex), and had found it to be helpful and well-tolerated. She could not recall why it had been stopped. She was aware of the birth defect hazards and was protected against pregnancy. Accordingly, she was advised to stay off the AAP, and was re-started on divalproex, and the problem was resolved.

These cases illustrate some important **diagnostic** points:

- Severe, disruptive anxiety may be a third but little-described presentation of mania (after the more commonly expected irritable/explosive and euphoric/ top-of-the-world patterns).

- If the patient is felt to have a mood disorder (major depressive disorder or bipolar disorder), then severe, treatment-resistant anxiety points to bipolar disorder rather than major depressive disorder. Or, more simply, anxiety that has resisted prior treatments suggests the mood condition might not be depression, but rather bipolar disorder (specifically mania or mixed episode). Or, even more simply, treatment-resistant anxiety suggests mania or mixed episode.

- As described in the prior chapter, if the patient's symptom description includes depression, it is important to ask the patient to explain in more detail exactly what it is that they're experiencing.

- As described in Chapter 6, it is crucial to find out just how many hours the patient is sleeping per night over the past week, because the highly anxious patient is also often having trouble sleeping. If a known bipolar patient[w] is sleeping less than 6 hours per night (despite having the opportunity to do so), this for all practical purposes rules out pure bipolar depression, and one is instead dealing with a manic or mixed episode.

These cases also illustrate some important points about bipolar disorder **treatment**:

If the responding clinician in Case 17.2 had taken Mrs. N's complaint of "severe anxiety" at face value, a simple but large increase in the patient's benzodiazepine anti-anxiety medication might have been of some help, say an increase from the prior Ativan (lorazepam) 0.5 mg twice a day to an increased dose of 1.0 mg three or four times a day,

but…

- Using routine anti-anxiety medications such as the benzodiazepines (BZs) to treat mania, including the anxiety associated with mania, is like trying to ward off a charging rhinoceros with a fly-swatter. The BZs are sedating and thus may decrease one's safety when driving or operating dangerous machinery, etc. If the patient is vulnerable to addictions, the BZs may substantially

---

w Please note that insomnia is also fairly common in patients with unipolar disorder (major depressive disorder).

increase the risk of relapse into substance abuse. The BZs are not likely to worsen the mood disorder itself, but unfortunately they're also not likely to be very effective, that is, the mania will roll on largely unchanged,

which brings us to the next point…

- In bipolar patients,ˣ mood stabilizers are the best anti-anxiety medicines.ʸ

- In many but not all bipolar patients, very gradually reducing and stopping of antidepressants over a 6 to 12 month period under careful supervision of the treating clinician may be the second-best anxiety-reducing strategy related to medication.

- Careful, limited use of standard anti-anxiety medicines , such as the BZs, as add-ons may also be extremely helpful in the short term, but with the implementation of the two strategies immediately above, they tend to be less and less necessary over time.

This then often allows us to taper the patient off the standard anti-anxiety medicine, thereby allowing us to build a smaller, simpler, safer, and more compact regimen for ongoing treatment.[41] This is important to reduce the likelihood of drug interactions and excessive drowsiness or sluggishness from too many medicines. A smaller, simpler, more tolerable regimen also improves the odds that the patient will be willing to continue to take the medicines.

- As another possibility in Case 17.2, if the responding doctor had chosen to take Mrs. N's initial complaint of "severe anxiety and depression" at simple face value, she or he might have reasoned that the antidepressants, in

---

x as also in patients with severe personality disorders[155]

y Despite being tried on all the traditional mood stabilizers in the absence of antidepressants, some patients may not experience relief, and/or may not be able to tolerate the mood stabilizers. In such patients, a reasonable alternative is the atypical antipsychotics (AAPs) given with simultaneous as-needed side effect medicine for possible restlessness, such as Cogentin/benztropine, Benadryl/diphenhydramine, or others, given in the absence of antidepressants.

particular the SSRI and SNRI antidepressants, are very often effective for both anxiety and depression, and therefore added one of these,

but…

- In so doing, they might have failed to inquire further and discover the manic symptoms including shortened and broken sleep, racing thoughts, impulsivity and irritability, leading to serious interference with her functioning.

The situation where antidepressants are effective for both anxiety and depression is in major depressive disorder, not in bipolar disorder. With the patient currently in mania, there is no convincing evidence in the literature that this intervention of adding an SSRI or SNRI antidepressant would have any chance of helping, but it would have a pretty good chance of being associated over time with worsening of the patient's condition, including a significant chance of being associated over time with worse depression.

This may seem hard to imagine, so look it up in the references by Rosa, Bauer, and Eppel[12,25,26] in the References section at the back of the book. Then Google **Pub Med**, enter the authors' names from one of the articles, scroll down to the specific article, listed by year, and click on it. Pub Med often has an **abstract**, i.e., a summary of the article. Your local librarian may be able to get you the full article if you want.

The bottom lines:

Look very carefully for mania before treating depression and anxiety (see Chapter 12).

Treatment-resistant anxiety in mood patients involves over-activation, and thus suggests mania or mixed state.[44,204]

Severe anxiety may be a fairly common, but thus far largely overlooked, third presentation of mania.

In bipolar patients, mood stabilizers are the most effective anti-anxiety medications.

Section E:

Understanding Bipolar Disorder in Three Dimensions

Dimension I, the Long View Over Time, is discussed at length in Chapters 4, 5, 8, and 9.

The explanation of Dimension II, the Top-Down, Vertical View, is in Chapter 12.

Dimension III, the view Across the Spectrum(s) of Bipolar Disorders, Depressive Disorders, and Related Disorders (the Horizontal View), follows in Chapters 18 and 19.

Chapter 18

Horizontal View: The Full Spectrum of the Bipolar Disorders and the Highly Recurrent Mood Disorders

The horizontal spectrum view of bipolar disorder is usually presented in a horizontal graphic as follows:

Figure 18.1

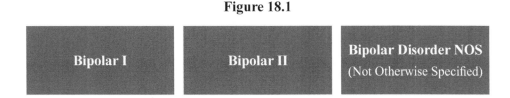

Unfortunately, this kind of graphic only tells somewhat less than half the story. In order to understand how bipolar disorder fits into the more interesting symphonic landscape of mood disorder, we must view it on a richer palette with a broader sweep.

Let's look at the wider sweep from the bipolar disorders through the unipolar disorders. This is shown in Figure 18.2 as a long horizontal sweep from left to right across the page, beginning with the most clearly bipolar disorder, bipolar I, then moving to the right through the less severe and less clearly bipolar disorders, to the junction between bipolar disorders and unipolar disorders at highly recurrent depression (HRUD). We then proceed through the most distinctly unipolar disorders, recurrent major depression, then further right through the less severe and less distinct unipolar disorders, clear through to the personality disorders, which are not really even unipolar disorders, but which nonetheless present with many depressing or discouraging situations, and with some depressive symptoms.

Figure 18.2, Full Horizontal Mood Spectrum

So, Good Heavens, you ask, what are all these things?? To answer, we'll work from left to right in Figure 18.2:

Bipolar I is the most obvious and severe form of bipolar disorder, with a full manic or mixed episode at some point during the course of the illness, which lasts at least 1 week (or any duration if hospitalization is needed, or psychosis occurs), and causes serious damage to work or social functioning. The episode(s) may be irritable or euphoric. Depressive episodes are not required for the diagnosis,[24] but are usually present nonetheless. (For more complete descriptions of these disorders, please see the Glossary and Appendix at the back of the book.)

Bipolar II disorder requires at least 1 episode very similar to a full manic episode, but less severe and less damaging. This is described as a "hypomanic" episode, that is, a minor manic episode. To qualify as a hypomanic episode under DSM-IV-TR[24] it must last at least 4 days, but it does not cause marked disruption of social or work functioning. To qualify as having bipolar II disorder, the patient must also have had at least 1 major depressive episode.[24]

Bipolar Disorder NOS (Not Otherwise Specified) is a disorder with similar manic, hypomanic, and/or mixed symptoms, but of shorter duration, and/or less severity than those described for bipolar I or II.[24]

Cyclothymia is a cycling bipolar disorder with numerous minor manias and minor depressions for 1 to 2 years, and with significant distress or social or work impairment.[24]

Highly Recurrent Unipolar Depression (HRUD, sometimes referred to as "cycling depression") has recurring unipolar depressive episodes, but essentially no manic or mixed symptoms. Some of its clinical features, including frequent cycling, seem to fall in between those of bipolar disorder and those of other recurrent major depressions.[174,177]

Another surprising thing is, even though it is by symptoms a unipolar disorder (depressions only, major depressive disorder[24]), HRUD often responds poorly to conventional/unipolar antidepressants, and responds as well or better in some studies, and in some cases in clinical practice, to the mood stabilizers lithium[175,176,177] or lamotrigine. In other words, HRUD is unipolar, but it sometimes seems to respond to treatment with medications as if it were bipolar.

Thus highly recurrent depression is the almost completely forgotten link between unipolar disorders and bipolar disorders, and it's important enough to be the subject of the next chapter, Chapter 19. As shown in Figure 18.2 above, a significant portion of patients with HRUD may fall into the broad category of bipolar spectrum disorders.[159,180]

Next as we move from left to right is Low Recurrence Unipolar Depressions, or LRUD.[174] This is a much more varied group of unipolar depressive disorders, including some with situational and personality features, rather than just pure mood disorder illnesses.[177,178]

Recurrent major depression is the current DSM-IV-TR[24] category which includes both HRUD and LRUD (See Figure 18.2 above), but DSM-IV-TR doesn't mention either one of these disorders specifically, that is, DSM-IV-TR makes no distinction between the two.

Major depression, single episode, is simply that, a single episode of significant depression lasting 2 weeks or more.

Depressive disorder NOS (Not Otherwise Specified), is a more vague grab bag of some noticeable depressive stuff, but without any full major depressive episodes.

Dysthymia is a chronic smoldering depression of 2 or more years duration, that never meets full major depression criteria. Surprisingly, however, some studies have shown dysthymia to cause just as much life disruption as major depression. Dysthymia precedes major depression in the life history of some individual patients, and this may then be referred to as "double depression."

Adjustment disorder is a condition involving excessive or disruptive reactions to various "stressors,"[24] i.e., upsetting situations or events. The reactions often include down or depressed feelings. They may not require treatment, and they may be more likely to respond to psychotherapy (talk therapy) than to medication or other medical treatments.

Personality disorder is a collection of disorders which are essentially lifelong, ineffective, maladaptive, or self-defeating reactions to various real and perceived childhood and ongoing situational insults. Personality disorders may be related to childhood trauma, and these people live very stressful, unhappy lives for which they tend to blame others or external circumstances. As a result, they often do not respond well to treatment (see Glossary).

No medication treatment is consistently effective for personality disorders, but a large recent study of severe personality disorders found that mood stabilizers were significantly more effective than antidepressants and antipsychotic medications.[155]

We have now discussed the more complete spectrum from bipolar disorders through the unipolar disorders.

Next, we'll look at some of the history and mystery surrounding the largely forgotten link between bipolar disorders and unipolar disorders: highly recurrent unipolar depression.

Chapter 19

Highly Recurrent Unipolar Depression (HRUD, Frequent Depressions With No Manias): The Unipolar Disorder That Thinks It's Bipolar

(Or…The Forgotten Link Between Unipolar Disorder and Bipolar Disorder)

For some reason, I started to see a handful of patients with this disorder in the 2000s. Some had failed numerous standard treatments for depression, which would have been expected to work. I was vaguely familiar with the pattern from some lectures and discussions during my residency in the late 1970s and 1980. I recalled the disorder as "cycling depression," and that it was characterized by frequent moderate to severe depressive episodes without significant manic or hypomanic episodes. The episodes often had a more regular rhythm or cycling pattern as compared to other major depressive episodes (low recurrence unipolar depression, or LRUD), as shown in Figure 19.1 below:

Figure 19.1

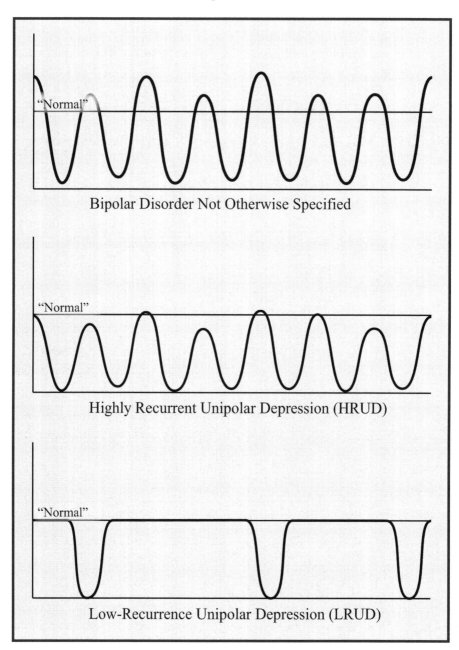

Bipolar Disorder Not Otherwise Specified

Highly Recurrent Unipolar Depression (HRUD)

Low-Recurrence Unipolar Depression (LRUD)

Accordingly, I treated the above patients with lithium or lamotrigine (Lamictal), the newest traditional mood stabilizer, which appears more effective for depressions than for manias, and the patients generally did well, but I was frustrated at how vague my recollection of the disorder was, and I couldn't find a subject file for it in my file cabinets, nor could I find out much about "cycling depression" in a cursory literature search.

So when I had the opportunity to attend the International Conference on Bipolar Disorders in Pittsburgh in 2007, I started asking mood experts who might be able to help me figure this out. Fortunately, a couple of folks knew what I was talking about, and steered me to Professor Guy Goodwin, who at the time was the chairman of the psychiatry department at Oxford. He explained that what I had been taught under the name of "cycling depression," was more commonly referred to as "highly recurrent depression" (referred to in this book as highly recurrent unipolar depression, or HRUD). He kindly sent me some helpful references on the disorder.

Studies from the past forty years, as reviewed by Frederick K. Goodwin and Kay Redfield Jamison,[4,177] and by Professor Guy Goodwin at Oxford, had surprisingly showed that this distinct pattern of depressions without manias nonetheless sometimes responded as well or better to lithium than to standard and well-proven unipolar antidepressant medicines.[175,176,191,198] In other words, this disorder looked unipolar (depression without mania), but its treatment response and some of its clinical features[174] were more similar to those one would expect with a bipolar disorder.

Interestingly enough, I recently discovered a 2005 study of maintenance treatment in rapid-cycling bipolar disorder that claimed that "highly recurrent refractory depression may be the hallmark of rapid-cycling bipolar disorder."[179] That is, as also discussed in Chapters 4 and 5, highly recurrent depression is one of the known clinical pictures of late course bipolar disorder, and so this may look very much like highly recurrent **unipolar** depression!

If the clinician in such a case failed to get the full lifetime history of mood episodes, they might easily see a new patient with frequent depressive spells and no recent manias, and conclude the patient was suffering unipolar disorder (major depressive disorder), when instead the patient was actually suffering rapid-cycling depressive episodes as part of late course bipolar disorder.

In summary, although I'd been a mood disorders specialist for over 10 years at the time (2007), my recollection of HRUD was pretty vague. During that 10 years, I had never seen a journal article about this disorder, and I had never heard a colleague mention it.

An example follows as to how the HRUD concept helped one patient and I in the process of understanding her mood disorder:

Case 19.1: Mrs. V consulted me in her late 40s with a history of many years of depression treated by primary doctors and psychiatrists with a series of 8 different antidepressants, none of which had helped. One of them, Wellbutrin/bupropion had made her extremely irritable. Six of them had been so poorly tolerated they had to be stopped. She came to me on the most recent antidepressant, Lexapro/escitalopram at 10 mg/day, and noted that this one had previously lost effectiveness ("pooped out") after 1 year. Mrs. V had no clear symptoms of over-activation or mania. I had her fill out a Mood Disorder Questionnaire[55] as part of the initial evaluation screening for possible bipolar disorder, and her responses gave no hint of manic or mixed symptoms. She was therefore initially felt to have recurrent major depression (unipolar disorder), which would fit with the bottom mood tracing in Figure 19.1, LRUD.

Accordingly, we tried increasing her Lexapro to the generally more effective dose of 20 mg/day, but she then experienced worse irritability, along with some increase in racing thoughts, distractibility, mood swings, and feeling racy and "wound up." We therefore decreased her Lexapro to 15 mg/day and eventually back to 10 mg/day.

I asked her for some more specific description of the pattern of her depressive mood swings. (I often do this by having patients compare their mood symptom patterns with the mood curves in Figure 19.1 [without the diagnostic labels attached].) She described a pattern most consistent with HRUD, the middle mood diagram in Figure 19.1.

She had never had a trial of a mood stabilizer, so, based on my awareness of the response patterns seen with HRUD, we added lithium to the Lexapro, and she showed significant improvement, but she couldn't tolerate the lithium side effects. We therefore decided to switch from the lithium to the AAP Abilify/

aripiprazole.[z]

We started at 2 mg/day of Abilify, and Mrs. V noted steady and significant improvement in symptoms over the next 3 to 4 months. Each dose increase brought further improvement all the way up to 15 mg/day. She felt as if she was likely to improve further at even higher doses.

This is somewhat noteworthy in that this dose is at the upper limit of the dose range recommended as an add-on treatment for treatment-resistant major depression (2 to 15 mg/day), and just at the lower end of the range of doses found to be effective for manic and mixed bipolar disorder in the FDA registration trials of Abilify (that is, 15 or 30 mg/day).

One of the most prominent symptoms the Abilify seemed to help was her irritability, a symptom she had mentioned repeatedly as occurring together with her depression, so I asked her how old she was when she had first experienced the depression together with significant irritability. Mrs. V then told me that these mixed spells of depression with irritability began at age 15 as brief 1 to 2-day spells, and as the first depressions she had ever experienced.

She continued to experience these ever after, alternating with longer depressive spells without the irritability. By this point her pattern of mood symptoms and responses to antidepressants and antimanic medicines (lithium and Abilify) appeared to have some of the features of the top mood picture in Figure 19.1, bipolar disorder not otherwise specified, so we tried reducing the Lexapro further down to 5 mg/day, with a further slight reduction in irritability and no recurrence of depression.

With the above medication changes over about seven months of treatment, including first adding lithium, then switching from lithium to Abilify, and with the reduction of her Lexapro, her condition had improved substantially compared to when she first saw me. She now felt the best she had since she was in her 20s, some 25 years earlier.

The above case illustrates how understanding the broader range of mood disorders can substantially improve outcomes for certain patients. Highly

---

z Abilify/aripiprazole has been FDA-approved as an acute treatment of manic or mixed episodes, as a maintenance treatment of bipolar disorder, and also as an add-on to antidepressants for treatment-resistant major depressive disorder, that is, it would cover any of the disorders we were considering as possiblities.

recurrent depression (HRUD), as well as its links to neighboring disorders, has been almost entirely forgotten, aside from a few mood disorders specialists. Given the stark difference between the clearly unipolar presentation of HRUD and the entirely different treatment response, one would suspect that this disorder possibly accounts for thousands of treatment failures, thereby unnecessarily delaying the recovery of thousands of patients.

Section F:

Looking Forward

CALM SEAS

Chapter 20

The Goal

We have the opportunity to help 5 million people,
patients with bipolar disorder
and their families and loved ones,
to achieve a substantially higher quality of life.

There are approximately 310 million people in the United States alone,[217] of whom approximately 3% to 4%[1,45,55,183] suffer with bipolar disorder. That's about 10 million people with bipolar disorder. Perhaps half of them are getting some form of treatment, which would be 5 million individuals.

By any information I have been able to find so far, at least half of these people fail to reach stable recovery, that is, about 2.5 million people. The illness and its effects have seriously damaged the life quality of at least 1 other person aside from the patient, and usually far more than that, and so, between the patients and those close to them, the number of people who stand to benefit substantially from an improvement in the real-world applied treatment of bipolar disorder is at least 5 million people. It is this group whose quality of life we aim to improve.

How To Reach It:
Other Goals Along the Way / Ways to Get There:

This book is a guidebook for patients and their families and loved ones, to explain the findings of the scientific literature in a way that most people can understand, and with enough references so you can look things up and decide for yourself.

In the following paragraphs, "we" refers to all of us reading this book. Together we can make quite a difference and move much closer to achieving the goal of substantially improving the quality of life of 5 million people, including bipolar patients and their families and loved ones. Some of the ways to do this are as follows:

1. We, and those we know and care about, need to be well informed about bipolar disorder and its treatment. We can start by looking up things that affect our treatment and our outcomes on the DBSA (Depression and Bipolar Support Alliance) website, www.dbsalliance.org, or on Dr. Jim Phelps' website, www.psycheducation.org, or on our website, www.calmseas.us.
Read Dr. Jim Phelps' 2006 book, *Why Am I Still Depressed?*, and this book.

2. We need to develop stronger support systems and networks for patients and their loved ones. One of the keys to this is patient advocacy and support groups such as DBSA (Depression and Bipolar Support Alliance) and NAMI (National Alliance for the Mentally Ill).

Consider starting your own local chapter of DBSA or NAMI, or start attending their meetings if there are already established chapters in your area.

Work with DBSA and NAMI to empower their members and families and close support people to collaborate with their treating healthcare providers in such a way as to realistically expect and achieve better clinical outcomes for patients with bipolar disorder.

Support DBSA and NAMI in their grant-seeking and lobbying efforts to secure funding for research studies of bipolar disorder, training for clinicians in the diagnosis and treatment of bipolar disorder, public information campaigns, etc.

3. In order to reach the very achievable goal of much better outcomes and quality of life for 5 million people, awareness of bipolar disorder and successful treatment approaches needs to go viral. So if you find any of the above resources

helpful, pass them on to others you know who might find them helpful, and encourage them to pass them on to the next wave of people who might benefit. Consider passing whatever you find helpful on to those in your address book or e-mail contact list or social media network who would be likely to benefit.

4. We need to reach out to, engage, and increase the awareness of the clinician/ provider community of the more successful concepts, principles, and treatment approaches described here. This may be most effectively pursued together with support groups such as DBSA and NAMI.

Please note that these more successful approaches have been almost completely forgotten in the past 10 years. Most clinicians trained within the last 10 years haven't yet been informed of them and/or haven't been provided adequate training in their everyday clinical application.[8,9,92,93]

As a result, the approach of relying primarily on antidepressants and antipsychotics in the treatment of bipolar disorder is heavily dominant here in the United States,[8,9,92,93] and the associated rate of treatment failure is very high.[10,13,16,18,19,20,21,25,26,27,28,29,37,38,39,40,41,42,58,60,63,64,65,66,68,210]

This has heightened the stigma of bipolar disorder by leading many to believe that bipolar disorder is complex beyond anyone's ability to understand, and difficult to treat, or perhaps even altogether untreatable.

Fortunately, nothing could be further from the truth. Bipolar disorder does have some interesting complexity, but it can be learned and understood fairly easily. Much of it is explained clearly in this one small book. Much of the rest of it can be understood from Dr. Jim Phelps' book.

And far from being untreatable, bipolar disorder is extremely treatable, if one simply adheres to proven approaches. It would seem to me to be time once again that we teach these proven approaches to our psychiatric residents and psychiatric nurse practitioner candidates, and the Calm Seas group will be happy to assist in this process in whatever way we can.

As part of the above efforts, we need to help clinicians come to expect and achieve better outcomes in collaboration with their bipolar patients and families. One possible next step along the way is a clinician's version of this book with more detail about evidence-based successful treatment approaches and specifics as to how to implement them.

5. The www.calmseas.us. team plans to develop the information contained in this book in all formats helpful to patients, their families and close support people, and clinicians, and to provide this via our website as soon as it is available.

Over time, the www.calmseas.us. team plans to develop for clinicians a full user-friendly on-line course of study in bipolar disorder, complete with self-assessment measures. Our eventual aim is to issue certificates to those who successfully complete the course of study.

We need to train as many as 500 to 1,000 clinicians highly knowledgeable about bipolar disorder and its successful treatment. Such clinicians with specialized knowledge about bipolar disorder are urgently needed, and are currently in short supply.

Depending on the response, the above efforts might lead to the formation of a bipolar disorders academy or institute, such as The J. Patrick Duffy, M.D., Center for Bipolar Disorder and Clinical Excellence, with the hope of furthering the knowledge and skills of clinicians in diagnosing and treating bipolar disorder. If the opportunities arise, we might also establish a foundation to support the efforts of the Duffy Center to improve treatment outcomes and quality of life for those suffering with bipolar disorder.

6. We see poor outcomes in the treatment of bipolar disorder as compared to outcomes in other disorders, and poor outcomes compared to those achieved in other countries.[12,21,210] We also see poor outcomes compared to the readily achievable moderate to good outcomes with the use of long-known effective approaches.

Because of this, in my opinion, there should be a psychiatric subspecialty for bipolar disorder. This subspecialty would have specialized training programs, and full accreditation and subspecialty board examinations from the American Board of Psychiatry and Neurology. Thus far, there has been little support for this idea, but I will be actively listening with others in the field to hear whether there is a change in the level of interest.

In the meantime, however, I hope to be working with others to develop teaching and self-examination materials consistent with the high standards of the subspecialty boards for those who wish to test their knowledge in this way.

Please hold in your thoughts and prayers the 5 million people for whom a substantially improved quality of life is achievable, but not yet achieved.

Thank you very much for your interest and attention in reading this book. Please contact our website with additional ideas you may have about how we can reach the goal at www.calmseas.us.

CALM SEAS

Glossary and Abbreviations

(For more complete descriptions of psychiatric disorders, see the Appendix following this Glossary, or the DSM-IV-TR.[24])

AAPs – Atypical Anti-Psychotics (sometimes also referred to as Second-Generation Antipsychotics [SGAs]). These are the newer antipsychotics, such as clozapine (Clozaril), risperidone (Risperdal), olanzapine (Zyprexa), quetiapine (Seroquel and Seroquel XR), aripiprazole (Abilify), ziprasidone (Geodon), paloperidone (Invega), asenapine (Saphris), iloperidone (Fanapt), lurasidone (Latuda), and others, including possibly loxapine (Loxitane). They appear to be more effective, and are used much more frequently in bipolar disorder than the older Typical Antipsychotics, such as haloperidol (Haldol), chlorpromazine (Thorazine), fluphenazine (Prolixin), trifluoperazine (Stelazine), and perphenazine (Trilafon).

Activation – This refers to the level of energy and activity, and it is important because along with Hours of Sleep per 24 Hours, it is one of the most reliable ways of determining whether a bipolar patient is in a state of mania, mixed episode, or depression. It is much more reliable than reported mood, for instance (See Chapters 5, 6, and 16).

Adjustment Disorder – A stress-related disturbance that lasts no more than 6 months, but causes marked distress or significant impairment in social or occupational functioning.

ADs – Anti-Depressants, as in regular or conventional or "unipolar" antidepressants. These work pretty well for major depressive disorder[24] (depressions with no manias, hypomanias, or mixed states, ever), but seem to help only 1 in 6 bipolar patients with depression.

179

BADs – See Bipolar Antidepressants below.

BCN – Bipolar Collaborative Network, see SFBN/BCN

Benzodiazepines – BZs, such as lorazepam (Ativan), clonazepam (Klonopin), alprazolam (Xanax), and diazepam (Valium). These are antianxiety medications with some addictive risk.

Big Three Mood Stabilizers – This refers to the traditional mood stabilizers lithium (Eskalith CR, LithoBID, and others), divalproex (Depakote and Depakote ER), and carbamazepine (Equetro, Tegretol, Carbatrol, and others).

Bipolar Antidepressants (BADs) – These agents, currently including lamotrigine (Lamictal), quetiapine (Seroquel XR), lithium, olanzapine (Zyprexa), and possibly lurasidone (Latuda), have demonstrated effectiveness in the treatment of bipolar depression. They are overall less effective in unipolar disorder/major depressive disorder.

Bipolar I Disorder – Bipolar I is the most obvious and severe form of bipolar disorder. It requires a full manic or mixed episode, which lasts at least 1 week (or any duration if hospitalization is needed or psychosis occurs [loss of touch with reality]), and causes serious damage, i.e., relationship loss, job loss, severe financial damage (e.g., from serious out-of-control spending), high-risk behavior (e.g., dangerous driving, speeding leading to arrests or accidents, or reckless promiscuity), psychiatric hospitalization, or (psychosis). Manias may be irritable or euphoric. Depressive episodes are not required for the diagnosis,[24] but are usually present.

Bipolar II Disorder – has at least 1 very similar but less severe, i.e., minor manic ("hypomanic") episode that lasts at least 4 days and has less severe and less damaging consequences than those noted above for bipolar I disorder. At least 1 major depressive episode is also required as part of bipolar II disorder.[24]

Bipolar Disorder NOS (Not Otherwise Specified) – a disorder with similar manic, hypomanic, and/or mixed symptoms, but of shorter duration, and/or less severity than those described for bipolar I or II.[24]

Bipolar Spectrum Disorders – Bipolar disorder NOS, cyclothymia, and highly recurrent unipolar depression / HRUD (see Chapter 18, esp. Figure 18.2).

BZs – See Benzodiazepines.

Carbamazepine – Carbamazepine is the generic compound found in the brand medicines Equetro, Tegretol, Carbatrol, Tegretrol XR, etc. Equetro, a controlled-release form of carbamazepine, is the only one with specific FDA-approval, in this case for the treatment of manic and mixed episodes.

Carbatrol – See Carbamazepine

Circadian Rhythms – Daily biological rhythms, including the sleep-wake cycle.

Clinician – Doctor or other healthcare provider or other prescriber (includes nurse practitioners, physicians' assistants, and others with authority to prescribe medicine for bipolar patients).

Correct Diagnosis – When I refer to bipolar disorder, it is generally assumed that the diagnosis was made in an thorough, careful, and accurate manner. Whenever this is in doubt, the patient needs to be fully re-evaluated, including taking a lifelong history of all mood episodes.

CRBBT – Cycling-and-Recurrence Based Bipolar Treatment. This approach focuses on cycling and recurrence as the main bipolar disorder features (rather than polarity). CRBBT relies most heavily on the mood stabilizers and tends to limit use of the antidepressants (see Chapter 3).

Cycling – This simply refers to the strong tendency in bipolar disorders and other mood disorders for activation, energy levels, and moods to cycle up and down. See also Rapid Cycling and Ultra-Rapid and Ultradian Cycling.

Cyclothymia – A cycling mood disorder lasting at least 1 to 2 years with mild manic episodes (hypomanic episodes) and mild depressive episodes, not meeting the criteria for full manic episode or full major depressive episode.[24]

Day-Night Reversal (D-N R): This occurs when the patient gets most of their sleep during the day, and most of their activity during the night. Unless their work requires this, for instance with policemen, firemen, nurses, etc., it should be avoided, as this is a serious problem that may interfere with recovery from bipolar disorder.

Depakene – See Divalproex.

Depakote, Depakote ER – See Divalproex.

Depression (only) – See Unipolar Disorder below.

Depressive Disorder NOS – Depressive disorder that doesn't meet criteria for any of the other specific DSM-IV-TR depressive disorders. Examples given include pre-menstrual dysphoric disorder, minor depressive disorder, and recurrent brief depressive disorder.[24]

Divalproex – Divalproex sodium is the generic compound of Depakote and Depakote ER, and is a form of valproic acid/valproate. Valproic acid itself is also used like divalproex, and is the generic compound found in Depakene.

DMX – Depressive mixed episode. A mixed episode or mixed state with more (or more severe) depressive than manic symptoms.

Doctor – The term doctor will be used to mean whoever is prescribing medicine. This term then may also stand for other clinicians who might be doing so, including nurse practitioners, physicians' assistants or other clinicians with prescribing privileges.

DSM, DSM-IV-TR – Diagnostic and Statistical Manual of the American

Psychiatric Association. Through May 2013, this has been the DSM-IV-TR: American Psychiatric Association (2000): *Diagnostic and Statistical Manual of Mental Disorders, Fourth Edition, Text Revision.* Washington, DC: American Psychiatric Association. (The next DSM after the DSM-IV-TR will be the DSM-5.)

Dysthymia – See Unipolar Disorder below. Dysthymic Disorder is a chronic smoldering unipolar depression that lasts at least 2 years, but never meets the criteria for a major depressive episode.

Early Course – In many patients, the first few years or first few episodes of bipolar disorder, characterized by simpler manic or depressive episodes. (See Chapter 4.) The early course of bipolar disorder may be skipped in many patients with childhood onset.

Equetro – See Carbamazepine.

FDA – Food and Drug Administration. This federal bureau decides on which medicines are approved for the treatment of specific medical disorders for marketing in the US.

Highly Recurrent Unipolar Depression – (HRUD, sometimes referred to as "cycling depression") has unipolar phenomena, i.e., recurring depressive episodes, but essentially no clear manic or mixed symptoms. Some of its clinical features, including frequent cycling, seem to fall in between those of bipolar disorder and those of other recurrent major depressions (See Chapters 18 and 19).[174,177]

Hours of Sleep per 24 Hours – This is just what it says, and may be abbreviated as a number, or range of numbers, over a slash, then 24: so for instance 7/24 would be 7 hours sleep per 24 hours, and 4-6/24 would mean 4 to 6 hours per 24 hours. The hours slept during the night sleep period are in some ways more important. If a patient's sleep is broken up between some at night and a daytime nap, we might abbreviate it as 6+2/24, say, for 6 hours at night and a

2 hour daytime nap. Hours of sleep per 24 hours is the single best marker of the current bipolar mood state, and this is described further in Chapter 6 on Duffy's Rule.

Hypomania – A somewhat less severe episode of mania (See DSM-IV-TR definition in the Appendix).

IPSRT – InterPersonal and Social Rhythm Therapy. This therapy focuses on developing "lifestyle regularity" as a way to stabilize circadian rhythms, including the sleep-wake cycle.

Lamotrigine – The original brand name is Lamictal. This is a mood stabilizer with weak anti-manic properties, but strong protection against future depressive episodes.

Late Course – In many patients, the late course begins after 5 mood episodes or 5 to 10 years of illness. Late course illness is characterized by rapid, ultra-rapid, or ultradian cycling, and by mixed episodes, which have manic and depressive symptoms co-occurring. In some patients with mixed episodes, the simultaneously occurring manic and depressive symptoms may swing up and down very rapidly, unpredictably, and entirely independently of each other, in what is described in Chapter 4 and Figure 4.4 as a rapidly shifting mixed episode (RSME).

Lithium – Lithium carbonate. This is the oldest and best-established mood stabilizer, having been discovered in 1949 by an Australian state hospital doctor with no research budget, in the hope that he could reduce deaths due to manic exhaustion. Brand names have included Eskalith, Eskalith CR, LithoBID, Lithonate, and others. It also comes as a liquid, lithium citrate.

Low Recurrence Unipolar Depression (LRUD) – See Unipolar Disorder below. This is a recurrent unipolar/major depressive disorder without frequent or highly regular recurrence, as in contrast to Highly Recurrent Unipolar Depression (HRUD).

Major Depression, Single Episode – See Unipolar Disorder below. This is simply a major depression of at least two weeks' duration, but with no recurrence.

Major Depressive Disorder – See Unipolar Disorder below.

MINI – Mini-International Neuropsychiatric Interview. Structured interview instrument that screens for **all the major psychiatric disorders** in a single interview generally lasting about an hour.[212]

MIX – Pure/DSM-IV-TR[24] mixed episode. This is a mixed episode with relatively severe manic symptoms and relatively severe depressive symptoms nearly every day during the same period of a week or longer.

Mixed Episodes / Mixed States – Mood episodes containing both manic and depressive symptoms. See also DMX, MIX, and MMX.

MMX – Manic mixed episode. A mixed episode or mixed state with more (or more severe) manic than depressive symptoms.

Mood Disorder Questionnaire (MDQ)[55] – This is a screening questionnaire developed by Robert Hirschfeld, M.D., of the University of Texas Medical Branch in Galveston. It is important that it be used in conjunction with a complete psychiatric evaluation.[85]

MSs – Mood Stabilizers. In this book this will refer to the four traditional mood stabilizers lithium (Eskalith, LithoBID, and others) , divalproex (Depakote and Depakote ER), carbamazepine (Equetro, Tegretol, Carbatrol, and others), and lamotrigine (Lamictal), although some other medicines, primarily the atypical antipsychotics, also possess mood-stabilizing properties, as may also possibly oxcarbazepine (Trileptal).

PBBT – Polarity-based bipolar treatment. This approach views short-term polarity as the most important treatment issue (rather than cycling and recurrence, see Chapter 3). PBBT relies heavily on the antidepressants, and often omits the traditional mood stabilizers.

Personality Disorder – a collection of disorders which are essentially lifelong, ineffective, maladaptive, or self-defeating behaviors, as well as feelings of "depression" or "stress," and unhappiness. Patients with personality disorders tend to view all the problems as being caused by others or external circumstances, and as a result these disorders may be very difficult to treat.

Polarity – This refers to whether mood states are up (manic) or down (depressed).
Prescriber – Same as Clinician above.

Psychiatric Resident – Medical doctor in the process of completing at least 4 years of additonal training beyond the M.D. or D.O. degree to become a psychiatrist, which is a medical specialist in psychiatry.

Psychosis – Significant loss of touch with reality, i.e., with hallucinations or delusions. Hallucinations involve perceiving things or people who aren't really there. These may occur in any sensation, but most commonly as voices or visions. Delusions are firmly held false beliefs, for instance when a person falsely believes they are a famous historical figure and have great powers, or when they feel they are under surveillance and likely attack by the Mafia or the CIA.

Rapid Cycling – Four or more illness episodes per year (total of the manic episodes and depressed episodes added together). See also Ultra-Rapid and Ultradian Cycling.

Rapidly Shifting Mixed Episode (RSME) – See also Figure 4.4. An ongoing mixed episode that includes extremely rapid shifts between mood states including manic and depressive symptoms. Patients in the midst of an RSME generally have **both manic and depressive symptoms of varying degrees** most days.

Recurrence – This simply refers to the fact that in mood disorders, including bipolar disorder, mood episodes or bouts of illness tend to come back again and again, even though they may be periodically separated by times of normal mood, energy, and activation.

Recurrent Major Depression – See Unipolar Disorder below.

"Regular Depression" – See Unipolar Disorder below.

Resident – See Psychiatric Resident, above.

RSME – See Rapidly Shifting Mood Episode above.

Severe Mood Dysregulation (SMD) – A childhood mood illness with **constant irritability**, as contrasted with childhood bipolar disorder, which would usually be expected to have episodic irritability.

SFBN, SFBN/BCN – The Stanley Foundation Bipolar Network, and its successor group, the Bipolar Collaborative Network, is a team of specialists at bipolar disorder research and treatment centers in the US and Europe. This group has carried out several important large-scale research studies, the results of which have been published in dozens of research and review articles, many of which are referenced in this book.

SMD – See Severe Mood Dysregulation above.

SNRIs – Serotonin and norepinephrine reuptake inhibitors, such as venlafaxine (Effexor), duloxetine (Cymbalta), and desvenlafaxine (Pristiq). These medicines are very similar to the very popular SSRIs, but due to their effect on norepinephrine, they may be somewhat more activating, and therefore somewhat more likely to precipitate mania or mixed states if given to patients with bipolar disorder.

SSRIs – Selective serotonin reuptake inhibitors, such as fluoxetine (Prozac), sertraline (Zoloft), paroxetine (Paxil), escitalopram (Lexapro), citalopram (Celexa), and fluvoxamine (Luvox). These medicines are effective for many anxiety disorders, and are the most commonly prescribed antidepressants. As with other antidepressants, however, they are not usually effective long-term in the treatment of patients with bipolar disorder.

STEP-BD – Systematic Treatment Enhancement Program for Bipolar Disorder. This research has been funded by the National Institutes of Mental Health (NIMH). STEP-BD is one of the largest multi-center series of research studies, and along with the SFBN-BCN, the most informative. STEP-BD studies are repeatedly referenced in this book.

Tegretol – See Carbamazepine above.

UADs – See Unipolar Antidepressants below.

Ultradian Cycling – Bipolar disorder late course mood cycling with multiple mood episodes within the same day[4,6] (Figure 4.3).

Ultra-Rapid Cycling, – Bipolar disorder late course mood cycling with multiple distinct mood episodes within a week[5] (as shown also in Figure 4.2)

Unipolar Disorder, or Unipolar Depression – This is major depressive disorder, which I refers to in some places as "regular depression," that is major depression without any significant manic, hypomanic, or mixed episodes, ever during the patient's entire life. If the patient ever has a serious manic, hypomanic or mixed episode, the diagnosis automatically changes to bipolar disorder for life.

The only exceptions to this rule are when other very major disorders are found to have provoked or mimicked the manic, hypomanic, or mixed symptoms. Examples include serious alcohol or drug abuse, obvious and overwhelming medical
or neurologic disorders, or schizophrenia.

Unipolar Antidepressants (UADs) – Conventional antidepressants, which are often effective in unipolar disorder/major depressive disorder. They are, however, only infrequently effective in bipolar disorder.

Valproic Acid – See Divalproex.

CALM SEAS

Appendix

Selected DSM-IV-TR Diagnostic Criteria[24] aa

I. Bipolar I Disorder requires the patient to
have had at least one Manic or Mixed Episode (See Criteria below).

Manic Episode

A. A distinct period of abnormally and persistently elevated, expansive, or irritable mood, lasting at least 1 week (or any duration if hospitalization is necessary).

B. During the period of mood distubance, three (or more) of the following symptoms have persisted (four if the mood is only irritable) and have been present to a significant degree:

(1) inflated esteem or grandiosity

(2) decreased need for sleep (e.g., feels rested after only 3 hours of sleep)

(3) more talkative than usual or pressure to keep talking

(4) flight of ideas or subjective experience that thoughts are racing

(5) distractibility (i.e., attention too easily drawn to unimportant or irrelevant external stimuli)

(6) increase in goal-directed activity (either socially, at work or school, or sexually) or psychomotor agitation

(7) excessive involvement in pleasurable activities that have a high potential for painful consequences (e.g., engaging in unrestrained buying sprees, sexual indiscretions, or foolish business investments)

C. The symptoms do not meet criteria for a Mixed Episode (see below).

---

aa Diagnostic Criteria in this Appendix reproduced with permission from the *Diagnostic and Statistical Manual of Mental Disorders, Fourth Edition, Text Revision* (Copyright 2000), American Psychiatric Association.

D. The mood disturbance is sufficiently severe to cause marked impairment in occupational functioning or in usual social activities or relationships with others, or to necessitate hospitalization to prevent harm to self or others, or there are psychotic features.

E. The symptoms are not due to the direct physiological effects of a substance (e.g., a drug of abuse, a medication, or other treatment) or a general medical condition (e.g., hyperthyroidism).

Note: Manic-like episodes that are clearly caused by somatic antidepressant treatment (e.g., medication, electroconvulsive therapy, light therapy) should not count toward a diagnosis of Bipolar I Disorder.

<u>Mixed Episode</u>

A. The criteria are met both for a Manic Episode (see above) and for a Major Depressive Episode (see below) (except for duration) nearly every day during at least a 1-week period.

B. The mood disturbance is sufficiently severe to cause marked impairment in occupational functioning or in usual social activities or relationships with others, or to necessitate hospitalization to prevent harm to self or others, or there are psychotic features.

E. The symptoms are not due to the direct physiological effects of a substance (e.g., a drug of abuse, a medication, or other treatment) or a general medical condition (e.g., hyperthyroidism).

Note: Mixed-like episodes that are clearly caused by somatic antidepressant treatment (e.g., medication, electroconvulsive therapy, light therapy) should not count toward a diagnosis of Bipolar I Disorder.

II. Bipolar II Disorder (Requires at least one
Major Depressive Episode and at least one Hypomanic Episode)

Hypomanic Episode

A. A distinct period of persistently elevated, expansive, or irritable mood, lasting throughout at least 4 days, that is clearly different from the usual nondepressed mood.

B. During the period of mood distubance, three (or more) of the following symptoms have persisted (four if the mood is only irritable) and have been present to a significant degree:
  (1) inflated esteem or grandiosity
  (2) decreased need for sleep (e.g., feels rested after only 3 hours of sleep)
  (3) more talkative than usual or pressure to keep talking
  (4) flight of ideas or subjective experience that thoughts are racing
  (5) distractibility (i.e., attention too easily drawn to unimportant or irrelevant external stimuli)
  (6) increase in goal-directed activity (either socially, at work or school, or sexually) or psychomotor agitation
  (7) excessive involvement in pleasurable activities that have a high potential for painful consequences (e.g., engaging in unrestrained buying sprees, sexual indiscretions, or foolish business investments)

C. The episode is associated with an unequivocal change in functioning that is uncharacteristic of the person when not symptomatic.

D. The disturbance in mood and the change in functioning are observable by others.

E. The episode is not severe enough to cause marked impairment in social or occupational functioning, or to necessitate hospitalization, and there are no psychotic features.

F. The symptoms are not due to the direct physiological effects of a substance (e.g., a drug of abuse, a medication, or other treatment) or a general medical condition (e.g., hyperthyroidism).

Note: Manic-like episodes that are clearly caused by somatic antidepressant treatment (e.g., medication, electroconvulsive therapy, light therapy) should not count toward a diagnosis of Bipolar II Disorder.

<u>Major Depressive Episode</u>

A. Five (or more) of the following symptoms have been present during the same 2-week period and represent a change from previous functioning; at least one of the symptoms is either (1) depressed mood or (2) loss of interest or pleasure.

   Note: Do not include symptoms that are clearly due to a general medical condition, or mood-incongruent delusions or hallucinations.

   (1) depressed mood most of the day, nearly every day, as indicated by either subjective report (e.g., feels sad or empty) or observation made by others (e.g., appears tearful).
   Note: In children and adolescents, can be irritable mood.
   (2) markedly diminished interest or pleasure in all, or almost all, activities most of the day, nearly every day (as indicated by either subjective account or observation made by others)
   (3) significant weight loss when not dieting or weight gain (e.g., a change of more than 5% of body weight in a month), or decrease or increase in appetite nearly every day.
   Note: In children, consider failure to make expected weight gains.
   (4) insomnia or hypersomnia nearly every day
   (5) psychomotor agitation or retardation nearly every day (observable by others, not merely subjective feelings of restlessness or being slowed down)
   (6) fatigue or loss of energy nearly every day

(7) feelings of worthlessness or excessive or inappropriate guilt (which may be delusional) nearly every day (not merely self-reproach or guilt about being sick)

(8) diminished ability to think or concentrate, or indecisiveness, nearly every day (either by subjective account or as observed by others)

(9) recurrent thoughts of death (not just fear of dying), recurrent suicidal ideation without a specific plan, or a suicide attempt or a a specific plan for committing suicide

B. The symptoms do not meet criteria for a Mixed Episode (see above).

C. The symptoms cause clinically significant distress or impairment in social, occupational, or other important areas of functioning.

D. The symptoms are not due to the direct physiological effects of a substance (e.g., a drug of abuse, a medication) or a general medical condition (e.g., hypothyroidism).

The symptoms are not better accounted for by Bereavement, i.e., after the loss of a loved one, the symptoms persist longer than 2 months or are characterized by marked functional impairment, morbid preoccupation with worthlessness, suicidal ideation, psychotic symptoms, or psychomotor retardation

III. Major Depressive Disorder, Recurrent

A. Presence of two or more Major Depressive Episodes (see above).

Note: To be considered separate episodes, there must be an interval of at least 2 consecutive months in which criteria are not met for a Major Depressive Episode.

B. The Major Depressive Episodes are not better accounted for by Schizoaffective Disorder and are not superimposed on Schizophrenia,

Schizophreniform Disorder, Delusional Disorder, or Psychotic Disorder Not Otherwise Specified.

C. There has never been a Manic Episode (see above), a Mixed Episode (see above), or a Hypomanic Episode (see above).

Note: This exclusion does not apply if all of the manic-like, mixed-like, or hypomanic-like episodes are substance or treatment induced or are due to the direct physiological effects of a general medical condition.

IV. Major Depressive Disorder, Single Episode

A. Presence of a single Major Depressive Episode (see above).

B. The Major Depressive Episode is not better accounted for by Schizoaffective Disorder and is not superimposed on Schizophrenia, Schizophreniform Disorder, Delusional Disorder, or Psychotic Disorder Not Otherwise Specified.

C. There has never been a Manic Episode (see above), a Mixed Episode (see above), or a Hypomanic Episode (see above).

Note: This exclusion does not apply if all of the manic-like, mixed-like, or hypomanic-like episodes are substance or treatment induced or are due to the direct physiological effects of a general medical condition.

References:

1. Merikangas KR, Akiskal JS, Angst J, et al. Lifetime and 12-month prevalence of bipolar spectrum disorder in the National Comorbidity Survey replication. Archives of General Psychiatry 2007; 64(5):543-552.

2. Michalak EE, Hole R, Holmes C, et al. Implications for psychiatric care of the word 'recovery' in people with bipolar disorder. Psychiatric Annals 2012; 42(5), p. 174.

3. Wisdom offered by one of my patients, 2012.

4. Goodwin FK, and Jamison KR (2007). *Manic-Depressive Illness: Bipolar Disorders and Recurrent Depression,* 2nd Edition. New York, NY: Oxford University Press.

5. Post RM, and Leverich GS (2008). *Treatment of Bipolar Illness: A Casebook for Clinicians and Patients.* New York, NY: W.W. Norton & Company.

6. Sachs GS (2004). *Managing Bipolar Affective Disorder* . London, UK: Science Press Ltd.

7. Ghaemi SN (2008). *Mood Disorders, A Practical Guide, Second Edition.* Philadelphia, PA: Wolters Kluwer Health.

8. Baldessarini RJ, Leahy L, Arcona S, et al. Patterns of psychotropic drug prescription for U.S. patients with diagnoses of bipolar disorders. Psychiatric Services 2007;58:85-91.

9. Baldessarini RJ, Henk H, Sklar A, et al. Psychotropic medications for patients with bipolar disorder in the United States: Polytherapy and adherence. Psychiatric Services 2008;59:1175-1183.

10. Altshuler L, Suppes T, Black D, et al. Impact of antidepressant discontinuation after acute bipolar depression remission on rates of depressive relapse at 1-year follow-up. American Journal of Psychiatry 2003; 160:1252-1262.

11. American Psychiatric Association: DSM-IV, *Diagnostic and Statistical Manual of Mental Disorders, Fourth Edition.* Washington DC: American Psychiatric Association, 1994.

12. Rosa AR, Cruz N, Franco C, et al. Why do clinicians maintain antidepressants in some patients with acute mania? Hints from the European Mania in Bipolar Longitudinal Evaluation of Medication (EMBLEM), a large naturalistic study. J Clin Psychiatry 2010;71(8):1000-1006.

13. Goldberg JF, Perlis RH, Ghaemi SN. Adjunctive antidepressant use and symptomatic recovery among bipolar depressed patients with concomitant manic

symptoms: findings from the STEP-BD. Am J Psychiatry 2007. 164(9):1348-1355.

14. Sparhawk R. Antidepressants in bipolar disorder: Caveats in interpreting and applying the finding of Altshuler et al. Journal of Clinical Psychiatry 2010; 71(2):211-212. The case vignette in Chapter 3, Case 3.1, was reproduced with the permission of Physicians Postgraduate Press, Inc.

15. Altshuler LL, Post RM, Hellemann G, et al. Impact of antidepressant continuation after acute positive or partial treatment response for bipolar depression: a blinded, randomized study. J Clin Psychiatry 2009; 70(4): 450-457.

16. Post RM, Leverich GS, Nolen WA, et al. A re-evaluation of the role of antidepressants in the treatment of bipolar depression: data from the Stanley Foundation Bipolar Network. Bipolar Disorders 2003; 5:396-406.

17. Post RM, Altshuler LL, Frye MA, et al. Complexity of pharmacologic treatment required for sustained improvement in outpatients with bipolar disorder. Journal of Clinical Psychiatry 2010; 71(9):1176-1186, page 1183.

18. Sachs GS, Nierenberg AA, Calabrese JR, et al. Effectiveness of adjunctive antidepressant treatment for bipolar depression. N Engl J Med 2007; 356(17):1711-1722.

19. Ghaemi SN, Ostracher MM, El-Mallakh RS, et al. Antidepressant discontinuation in bipolar depression: A Systematic Treatment Enhancement Program for Bipolar Depression (STEP-BD) randomized clinical trial of long-term effectiveness and safety. J Clin Psychiatry 2010; 71(4): 372-380.

20. Post RM, Altshuler LL, Frye MA, et al. Complexity of pharmacologic treatment required for sustained improvement in outpatients with bipolar disorder. Journal of Clinical Psychiatry 2010; 71(9):1176-1186.

21. Post RM, Leverich GS, Altshuler LL, et al. Differential clinical characteristics, medication usage, and treatment response in the US versus The Netherlands and Germany. Intl Clin Psychopharmacol 2011; 26(2):96-106.

22. Phelps J. Educating patients about bipolar disorders. Psychiatric Times, Jan 2012: pp. 33-38.

23. Phelps J. (2006). *Why Am I Still Depressed?, Bipolar II and Soft Bipolar Disorder.* New York, NY: McGraw Hill.

24. American Psychiatric Association (2000): *Diagnostic and Statistical Manual of Mental Disorders, Fourth Edition, Text Revision.* Washington, DC: American Psychiatric Association. See Appendix 1 for diagnostic criteria for manic episode, mixed episode, and hypomanic episode.

25. Bauer M, Rasgon N, Grof P, et al. Do antidepressants influence mood

patterns? a naturalistic study in bipolar disorder. Eur Psychiatry. 2006;21(4):262-269.

26. Eppel AB. Antidepressants in the treatment of bipolar disorder: decoding contradictory evidence and opinion. Harv Rev Psychiatry 2008;16:204-209.

27. Schneck CD, Miklovitz DJ, Miyahara S, et al. The prospective course of rapid-cycling bipolar disorder: findings from the STEP-BD. Am J Psychiatry 2008;165(3):370-377.

28. Sparhawk R. In bipolar disorder beyond 10 weeks of treatment, the term antidepressants is a misnomer (letter to the editor). J Clin Psychiatry 2011;72(6): 871.

29. Sidor MM and MacQueen GM. Antidepressants for the acute treatment of bipolar depression: a systematic review and meta-analysis. J Clin Psychiatry 2011;72(2):156-167.

30. Sachs, Gary, 2004. *Managing Bipolar Affective Disorder.* London, UK: Science Press. Chapter 1: Introduction to the Collaborative Care Model, pp. 1-22.

31. Ghaemi SN. Bipolar disorder and antidepressants: An ongoing controversy. Primary Psychiatry 2001; 8(2):28-34.

32. Goodwin FK and Jamison KR (2007). *Manic-Depressive Illness: Bipolar Disorders and Recurrent Depression, 2nd edition.* New York, NY: Oxford University Press, p. 31.

33. Sparhawk R and Ghaemi SN. CALM: A mnemonic for treatment options in bipolar disorder. Primary Care Companion to the Journal of Clinical Psychiatry 2008; 10(6): 485-486.

34. Goldberg JF, Garno IL, Leon AC, et al. Association of recurrent suicidal ideation with nonremission from acute mixed mania. Am J Psychiatry 1998; 155(12): 1753-1755.

35. Sato T, Bottlender R, Tanabe A, et al. Cincinnati criteria for mixed mania and suicidality in patients with acute mania. Compr Psychiatry 2004, Jan-Feb; 45(1): 62-69.

36. Ketter TA and Calabrese JR. Stabilization of mood from below versus above baseline in bipolar disorder: a new nomenclature. Journal of Clinical Psychiatry 2002; 63: 146-151.

37. Truman CJ, Goldberg JF, Ghaemi SN, et al. Self-reported history of manic/hypomanic switch associated with antidpressant use: data from the Systematic Treatment Enhancement Program for Bipolar Disorder (STEP-BE). J Clin Psychiatry 2007; 68:1472-1479.

38. Yerevanian BI, Koek RJ, Mintz J, et al. Bipolar pharmacotherapy and suicidal

behavior. Part 2. The impact of antidepressants. Journal of Affective Disorders 2007; 103:13-21.

39. Ghaemi SN, Wingo AP, Filkowski MA, et al. Long-term antidepressant treatment in bipolar disorder: meta-analysis of benefits and risks. Acta Psychiatrica Scandinavica 2008; 118(5): 347-356.

40. Ward, Christopher, 2012. *Balance.* Trafford Publishing, www. trafford.com. In this jarring first-person account of a patient with Bipolar I Disorder, note the periods of stability when he was treated briefly with lithium early on and again at the end. Then contrast these with the periods of extreme mood swings, crises, hospitalizations, inability to function right, etc., when he was treated instead with antidepressants.

41. Goldberg JF, Brooks JO, Kurita K, et al. Depressive illness burden associated with complex polypharmacy in patients with bipolar disorder: findings from the STEP-BD. J Clin Psychiatry 2009; 70(2): 155-162.

42. Leverich GS, Altshuler LL, Frye MA, et al. Risk of switch in mood polarity to hypomania or mania in patients with bipolar depression during acute and continuation of venlafaxine, sertraline, and bupropion as adjuncts to mood stabilizers. Am J Psychiatry 2006;163:232-239.

43. Sparhawk R, Ghaemi SN. Treatment strategies for bipolar disorder: CALM SEA. Primary Care Companion to the CNS Disorders 2011;13(3): 10|01106:e1-2.

44. Sparhawk R (2013). *CALM SEAS, Keys to the Successful Treatment of Bipolar Disorder:* Chapters 4 and 5, The Natural History of Bipolar Disorder.

45. Kessler RC, Petukhova M, Sampson NA, et al. Twelve-month and lifetime morbid risk of anxiety and mood disorders in the United States. Int J Methods Psychiatr Res 2012; 21(3): 169-184.

46. Kramer PD, 1993. *Listening to Prozac.* New York, NY: Penguin Books.

47. Zimmerman P, Brueckl, T, Nocon A, et al. Heterogeneity of DSM-IV major depressive disorder as a consequence of subthreshold bipolarity. Arch Gen Psychiatry, 2009; 66(12)1341-1352.

48. Angst J, Cui L, Swendsen J, et al. Major depressive disorder with subthreshold bipolarity in the National Comorbidity Survey Replication. Am J Psychiatry 2010; 167:1194-1201.

49. Stahl SM. S*tahl's Essential Psychopharmacology, Third Edition.* New York, NY: Cambridge University Press, Mood Disorders and Mood Stabilizers, pp 461-473 and 667-719.

50. Moreno C, Laje G, Blanco C, et al. National trends in the outpatient diagnosis and treatment of bipolar disorder in youth. Arch Gen Psychiatry 2007; 64(9):1032-

1039.

51. Frei R. Popularity of bipolar diagnosis in children and adolescents raises concerns. CNS News, March 2007, p. 22.

52. Blader JC, Carlson GA. Increased rates of bipolar disorder diagnoses among U.S. child, adolescent, and adult inpatients, 1996-2004. Biol Psychiatry 2007; 62(2): 107-114.

53. Leibenluft E. Severe mood dysregulation, irritability, and the diagnostic boundaries of bipolar disorder in youths. Am J Psychiatry 2011; 168:129-142.

54. Goodwin FK, and Jamison KR (2007). *Manic-Depressive Illness: Bipolar Disorders and Recurrent Depression, 2nd Edition.* New York, NY: Oxford University Press, pp 120-125.

55. Hirschfeld RM, Calabrese JR, Weissman MM, et al. Screening for bipolar disorder in the community. Journal of Clinical Psychiatry 2003; 64(1): 53-59.

56. Ritter PS, Marx C, Bauer M, et al. The role of disturbed sleep in the early recognition of bipolar disorder: a systematic review. Bipolar Disorders 2011; 13(3):227-237. (Review article with 69 further references.)

57. Berk M, Brnabic A, Dodd S, et al. Does stage of ilness impact treatment response in bipolar disorder? Empirical treatment data and their implication for the staging model and early intervention. Bipol Disord 2011; 13: 87-98.

58. Agren H, Backlund L. Bipolar disorder: Balancing mood states early in the course of illness effects long-term prognosis. Physiology and Behavior 2007; 92:199-202.

59. Undurraga J, Baldessarini RJ, Valenti M, et al. Suicidal risk factors in bipolar I and II disorders. J Clin Psychiatry 2012; 73(6): 778-782.

60. Post RM, Leverich GS, Altshuler LL, et al. Relationship of prior antidepressant exposure to long-term prospective outcome in bipolar I disorder outpatients. J Clin Psychiatry 2012; 73(7): 924-930.

61. Sparhawk R. Treatment of mood disorders: a surprising omission, and the role of lamotrigine as a prototypical bipolar antidepressant. Primary Psychiatry 2010;17(7):17-19.

62. Gan Z, Diao F, Wei Q, et al. A predictive model for diagnosing bipolar disorder based on the clinical characteristics of major depressive episodes in Chinese population. Journal Affective Disorders 2011; 134(1-3): 119-125.

63. Lish J, Dim-Meenan S, Whybrow PC, et al. The National Depressive and Manic-Depressive Association (DMDA) survey of bipolar members. J Affect Disord 1994;31:281-294.

64. Hirschfeld RM, Lewis L, Vornik LA. Perceptions and impact of bipolar

disorder: how far have we really come? Results of the National Depressive and Manic-Depressive Association 2000 survey of individuals with bipolar disorder. J Clin Psychiatry, 2003; 64(2):161-174.

65. Ghaemi SN, Sachs GS, Chiou AM, et al. Is bipolar disorder still underdiagnosed? Are antidepressants overutilized? J Affect Disord 1999;52:135-144.

66. Ghaemi SN, Boiman EE, Goodwin FK. Diagnosing bipolar disorder and the effects of antidepressants: a naturalistic study. J Clin Psychiatry 2000;61:804-808.

67. Symbyax product information, Physicians' Desk Reference, 59th Edition, 2005. Montvale NJ: Thomson PDR.

68. Frye MA, Helleman G, McElroy SL, et al. Correlates of treatment-emergent mania associated with antidepressant treatment in bipolar depression. Am J Psychiatry 2009; 166: 164-172.

69. Berk M, Berk L, Moss K, et al. Diagnosing bipolar disorder: How can we do it better? Med J Aust 2006; 184(9): 459-462

70. Chung H, Culpepper L, DeWester JN, et al. Challenges in diagnosing bipolar disorder: Identifying mixed episodes. Current Psychiatry, November 2006, Supplement S5-S10.

71. McElroy SL, Keck PE, Pope HG Jr, et al. Clinical and research implications of the diagnosis of dysphoric or mixed mania or hypomania. Am J Psychiatry 1992; 149: 1633-1644.

72. Goldberg JF, Perlis RH, Bowden CL, et al. Manic symptoms during depressive episodes in 1,380 pattients with bipolar disorder: Findings from the STEP-BD. Am J Psychiatry 2009; 166:173-181.

73. Goodwin FK, and Jamison KR (2007). *Manic-Depressive Illness: Bipolar Disorders and Recurrent Depression, 2nd Edition.* New York, NY: Oxford University Press, p. 72.

74. Faraone SV, Biederman J, Mennin D, et al. Is comorbidity with ADHD a marker for juvenile-onset mania? J Am Acad Child Adolesc Psychiatry 1997; 36: 1046-1055.

75. Geller B, Craney JL, Bolhofner K, et al. Two-year prospective follow-up of children with a prepubertal and early adolescent bipolar disorder phenotype. Am J Psychiatry 2002; 159: 927-933.

76. Geller B, Zimmerman B, Williams M, et al. DSM-IV mania symptoms in a prepubertal and early adolescent bipolar disorder phenotype compared to attention-deficit hyperactive and normal controls. J Child Adolesc Psychopharmacol 2002; 12: 11-25.

77. Goodwin FK, and Jamison KR (2007). *Manic-Depressive Illness: Bipolar Disorders and Recurrent Depression, 2nd Edition.* New York, NY: Oxford University Press, p. 31.

78. Kotin J, Goodwin FK. Depression during mania: Clinical observations and theoretical implications. Am J Psychiatry 1972; 129(6): 679-686.

79. Akiskal HS, Benazzi F, Perugi G, et al. Agitated "unipolar" depression re-conceptualized as depressive mixed state: implications for the antidepressant-suicide controversy. J Affect Disord 2005; 85(3): 245-248.

80. Benazzi F, Akiskal HS. Psychometric delineation of the most discriminant symptoms of depressive mixed states. Psychiatry Res 2006; 141: 81-88.

81. *Drug Facts and Comparisons 2004,* p. 1091. St. Louis, MO: Facts and Comparisons, part of Kluwer Health.

82. Post RM, Altshuler LL, Leverich GS, et al. Mood switch in bipolar depression: comparison of adjunctive venlafaxine, bupropion, and sertraline. British Journal of Psychiatry 2006; 189:124-131.

83. Torres IJ, DeFreitas VG, DeFreitas CM, et al. Neurocognitive functioning in patients with bipolar I disorder recently recovered from a first manic episode. Journal of Clinical Psychiatry 2010; 71(9): 1234-1242.

84. Ryan KA, Vederman AC, McFadden EM, et al. Differential executive functioning by phase of bipolar disorder. Bipolar Disorders 2012; 14: 527-536.

85. Zimmerman M. Misuse of the Mood Disorder Questionnaire as a case-finding measure and a critique of the concept of using a screening scale for bipolar disorder in psychiatric practice. Bipolar Disorders 2012; 14: 127-134.

86. Frank E, Hlastala S, Ritenour, et al. Inducing lifestyle regularity in recovering bipolar disorder patients: results from the maintenance therapies in bipolar disorder protocol. Biological Psychiatry 1997; 41: 1165-1173.

87. Geller B, Zimmerman B, Williams M, et al. Diagnostic characteristics of 93 cases of a prepubertal and early adolscent bipolar disorder phenotype by gender, puberty and comorid attention deficit hyperactivity disorder. J Child Adolesc Psychopharmacol 2000; 10: 157-164.

88. Gaedda GL, Baldessarini RJ, Glovinsky IP, et al. Pediatric bipolar disorder: phenomenology and course of illness. Bipolar Disord 2004; 6: 305-313.

89. Sparhawk R (2012). *CALM SEAS, Keys to Success in the Treatment of Bipolar Disorder:* Chapter 4, The Natural History of Bipolar Disorder.

90. Fardet L, Petersen I, Nazareth I, Suicidal behavior and severe neuropsychiatric disorders following glucocorticoid therapy in primary care. American Journal of Psychiatry 2012; 169: 491-497.

91. Ninth International Conference on Bipolar Disorder of the International Society for Bipolar Disorders, Pittsburgh, PA, June 2011.

92. Rakofsky JJ, Dunlop BW. US psychiatric residents' treatment of patients with bipolar disorder. Journal of Clinical Psychopharmacology 2012; 32(2):231-236.

93. "Is there a way to help residents become more comfortable with starting mood stabilizers, rather than rely on antipsychotics for mania?", a question written to me from two of the psychiatric residents attending the 9th International Conference on Bipolar Disorders, Pittsburgh, PA, June 2011.

94. Berk M, Dood S, Malhi GS. 'Bipolar missed states': the diagnosis and clinical salience of bipolar mixed states. Australian and New Zealand Journal of Psychiatry 2005; 39: 215-221.

95. Keck PE, Perlis RH, Otto MW, et al. Treatment of Bipolar Disorder 2004. Postgrad Med, Dec 2004 Special Report: 2-117.

96. Practice guideline for the treatment of patients with bipolar disorder (revision). American Journal of Psychiatry 2002; 159(4 Suppl):1-50.

97. Covey SR, 1989. *The Seven Habits of Highly Successful People.* Habit 2: Begin with the end in mind; pp. 95-144. New York, NY: Fireside/Simon & Schuster Inc.

98. Goodwin FK and Jamison KR, 2007. *Manic-Depressive Illness, Second Edition,* pp. 729-734.

99. Ghaemi SN, 2008. *Mood Disorders, Second Edition,* Practical Guides in Psychiatry, p.173. Philadelphia, PA: Wolters Kluwer.

100. Goodwin FK. Comment made frequently at continuing medical education seminars and noted by Ghaemi SN, 2008, in *Mood Disorders, Second Edition,* Practical Guides in Psychiatry, p.173. Philadelphia, PA: Wolters Kluwer.

101. Sachs GS. *Managing Bipolar Affective Disorder,* 2004. London, UK: Science Press Ltd., Chapter 6, Rapid Cycling Pathway, pp. 80-81.

102. Tohen M, Vieta E, Calabrese JR, et al. Efficacy of olanzapine and olanzapine-fluoxetine combination in the treatment of bipolar I depression. Archives of General Psychiatry 2003;60:1079-1088.

103. Calabrese JR, Bowden CL, Sachs G et al. A placebo-controlled 18-month trial of lamotrigine and lithium maintenance treatment in recently depressed patients with bipolar I disorder. J Clin Psychiatry 2003;64: 1013-1024.

104. Bowden CL, Calabrese JR, Sachs G et al. A placebo-controlled 18-month trial of lamotrigine and lithium maintenance treatment in recently manic or hypomanic patients with bipolar I disorder. Arch Gen Psychiatry 2003;60: 392-400.

105. Baldessarini RJ, Tondo L, Davis P, et al. Decreased risk of suicides during long-term lithium treatment: A meta-analytic review. Bipolar Disorders 2006; 8: 625-639.

106. Ghaemi SN. Hippocrates and Prozac: The controversy about antidepressants in bipolar disorder. Primary Psychiatry 2006; 13(11): 51-58, esp. "The pursuit of happiness."

107. Sachs GS. *Managing Bipolar Affective Disorder,* 2004. London, UK: Science Press Ltd., Rapid Cycling Pathway, Table 6.1, page 81. Dr. Sachs recommends a taper of 20-33% per month, which would work out to a taper period of 3-5 months.

108. National Institute for Health and Clinical Excellence (NICE), 2006. NICE Clinical Guideline on Bipolar Disorder in Adults, Children and Adolescents, in Primary and Secondary Care 2006; www.nice.org.uk/Guidance/CG38, accessed September 2012.

109. The Editors of American Heritage, adapted by Fred Cook, *The Golden Book of the American Revolution,* 1959. New York, NY: Golden Press, Inc., pp. 169-173.

110. Balazs J, Benazzi F, Rihmer Z, et al. The close link between suicide attempts and mixed (bipolar) depression: implications for suicide prevention. Journal of Affective Disorders 2006; 91: 133-138.

111. Young AH, Hammond JM. Lithium in mood disorders: Increasing evidence base, declining use? British Journal of Psychiatry 2007; 191: 474-476.

112. Blanco C, Laje G, Olfson M, et al. Trends in the treatment of bipolar disorder by outpatient psychiatrists. American Journal of Psychiatry 2002; 159(6): 1005-1010.

113. Yatham LN, Kennedy SH, Schaffer A, et al. Canadian Network for Mood and Anxiety Treatments (CANMAT) and International Society for Bipolar Disorders (ISBD) collaborative update of CANMAT guidelines for the management of patients with bipolar disorder: Update 2009. Bipolar Disorders 2009; 11(3): 225-255.

114. Bauer M, Ritter P, Grunze H, et al. Treatment options for acute depression in bipolar disorder. Bipolar Disorders, May 2012; Suppl 2: 37-50.

115. Jefferson JW. A clinician's guide to monitoring kidney function in lithium-treated patients. Journal of Clinical Psychiatry 2010; 71(9): 1153-1157.

116. Geddes JR, Goodwin GM, Rendell J, et al. Lithium plus valproate combination therapy versus monotherapy for relapse prevention in bipolar I disorder (BALANCE): a randomised open-label trial. Lancet 2010:; 375(9712): 385-395.

117. Kramer PD. *Listening to Prozac,* 1993. New York, NY: Penguin Books USA.

118. Pacchiarotti I, Nivoli AM, Mazzarini L, et al. The symptom structure of bipolar acute episodes: In search for the mixing link. Journal of Affective Disorders 2013, Feb 7, Epub ahead of print.

119. Rosenbaum CP and Beebe JE III (1975). *Psychiatric Treatment: Crisis, Clinic, and Consultation.* Chapter 11, Organizing Emergency Work, Part 2: Emergency Room Exercise, pp. 221-224. New York, NY: McGraw Hill, Inc.

120. American Psychiatric Association, 1980. *DSM-III, Diagnostic and Statistical Manual, Third Edition.* Washington DC: American Psychiatric Association.

121. Amsterdam JD, Shults J. Efficacy and safety of long-term fluoxetine versus lithium monotherapy of biolar II disorder: A randomized, double-blind, placebo-substitution study. American Journal of Psychiatry 2010; 167(7): 792-800.

122. Suppes T. Editorial: Is there a role for antidepressants in the treatment of bipolar II depression? American Journal of Psychiatry 2010; 167(7): 738-740.

123. Goodwin GM, Bowden CL, Calabrese JR, et al. A pooled analysis of 2 placebo-controlled 18-month trials of lamotrigine and lithium maintenance in bipolar I disorder. Journal of Clinical Psychiatry 2004; 65: 432-441.

124. Geddes JR, Calabrese JR, Goodwin GM. Lamotrigine for treatment of bipolar depression: Independent meta-analysis and meta-regression of individual patient data from five randomised trials. British Journal of Psychiatry 2009; 194(1): 4-9.

125. Zimmerman M, Galione JN, Ruggero CJ, et al. Screening for bipolar disorder and finding borderline personality disorder. Journal of Clinical Psychiatry 2010; 71(9): 1212-1217.

126. Tohen M, McDonnell DP, Case M, et al. Randomised, double-blind, placebo-controlled study of olanzapine in patients with bipolar I depression. British Journal of Psychiatry. Published online August 23, 2012. DOI: 10.1192/bjp.bp.112.108357.

127. Berk M, Hallam KT, McGorry PD. The potential utility of a staging model as a course specifier: A bipolar disorder perspective. Journal of Affective Disorders 2007; 100: 279-281.

128. Brown E, Dunner DL, McElroy SL, et al. Olanzapine/fluoxetine combination vs. lamotrigine in the 6-month treatment of bipolar I depression. International Journal of Nuropsychopharmacology 2009; 12: 773-782.

129. Strech D, Soltmann B, Weikert B, et al. Quality of reporting of randomized controlled trials of phamacologic treatment of bipolar disorders: A systematic

review. Journal of Clinical Psychiatry 2011; 72(9): 1214-1221.

130. Kupfer DJ, Frank E, Grochocinski VJ, et al. Demographic and clinical characteristics of individuals in a bipolar disorder case registry. Journal of Clinical Psychiatry 2002; 63(2): 120-125.

131. Baldessarini RJ, Vieta E, Calabrese JR, et al. Bipolar depression: Overview and commentary. Harvard Review of Psychiatry 2010; 18: 143-157.

132. Muzina DJ. Discontinuing an antidepressant? Tapering tips to ease distressing symptoms. Current Psychiatry 2010; 9(3): 51-61.

133. Post RM, and Leverich GS (2008). *Treatment of Bipolar Illness: A Casebook for Clinicians and Patients.* New York, NY: W.W. Norton & Company, Chapter 35, including A Sample Consultation About Alternative Treatment Approaches.

134. Phelps J. (2006). *Why Am I Still Depressed?, Bipolar II and Soft Bipolar Disorder.* New York, NY: McGraw Hill. Chapter 9: What you need to know when considering antidepressants.

135. Saunders KE, Goodwin GM. New approaches in the treatment of bipolar depression. Current Topics in Behavioral Neuroscience 2012 Aug 19 [Epub ahead of print].

136. Clark L, Iversen SD, Goodwin GM. Sustained attention deficit in bipolar disorder. British Journal of Psychiatry 2002; 180: 313-319.

137. Talbot LS, Stone S, Gruber J, et al. A test of the bidirectional association between sleep and mood in bipolar disorder and insomnia. Journal of Abnormal Psychology 2012; 121(1):39-50.

138. Akiskal HS, Benazzi F. Atypical depression: a variant of bipolar II or a bridge between unipolar and bipolar II? Journal of Affective Disorders 2005; 84: 209-217.

139. Frye MA, Yatham L, Ketter TA, et al. Depressive relapse during lithium treatment associated with increased serum thyroid-stimulating hormone: results from two placebo-controlled bipolar I maintenance studies. Acta Psychiatrica Sacandiinvavica 2009; 120: 10-13.

140. Lewis L. Patient perspectives on the diagnosis, treatment and management of bipolar disorder. Bipolar Disorders 2005; 7(Suppl. 1): 33-37.

141. Oquendo MA, Galfalvy HC, Currier D, et al. Treatment of suicide attempters with bipolar disorder: A randomized clinical trial comparing lithium and valproate in the prevention of suicidal behavior. American Journal of Psychiatry 2011; 168: 1050-1056.

142. Dias RS, Lafer B, Russo C, et al. Longitudinal follow-up of bipolar

disorder in women with premenstrual exacerbation: findings from the STEP-BD. American Journal of Psychiatry 2011; 168: 386-394.

143. Malhi GS, Adams D, Berk M. Medicating mood with maintenance in mind: bipolar depression pharmacotherapy. Bipolar Disorders 2009; 1(suppl 2): 55-76.

144. Frank E, Kupfer DJ, Thase ME, et al. Two-year outcomes for interpersonal and social rhythm therapy in individuals with bipolar I disorder. Archives of General Psychiatry 2005; 62(9): 996-1004.

145. Ghaemi SN. Why antidepressants are not antidepressants: STEP-BD, STAR*D, and the return of neurotic depression. Bipolar Disorders 2008; 10(8): 957-968.

146. Hantouche EG, Akiskal HS, Lancrenon S, et al. Systematic clinical methodology for validating bipolar-II disorder: Data in mid-stream from a French national multi-site study (EPIDEP). Journal of Affective Disorders 1998; 50: 163-173.

147. Dilsaver SC, Benazzi F, Akiskal HS. Mixed states: The most common outpatient presentation of bipolar depressed adolescents? Psychopathology 2005; 38(5): 268-272.

148. Yonkers KA, Wisner KL, Stowe Z, et al. Management of bipolar disorder during pregnancy and the postpartum period. American Journal of Psychiatry 2004; 161(4): 608-620.

149. Parekh PI, Ketter TA, Altshuler L, et al. Relationships between thyroid hormone and antidepressant responses to total sleep deprivation in mood disorder patients. Biological Psychiatry 1998; 43(5): 392-394.

150. Voderholzer U. Sleep deprivation and antidepressant treatment. Dialogues in Clinical Neuroscience 2003; 5(4): 366-369.

151. Sarris J, Mischoulon D, Schweitzer I. Omega-3 for bipolar disorder: Meta-analyses of use in mania and bipolar depression. Journal of Clinical Psychiatry 2012; 73(1): 81-86.

152. Koukopoulos A, Ghaemi SN. The primacy of mania: A reconsideration of mood disorders. Eur Psychiatry 2009; 24(2): 124-134.

153. Ehlers CL, Frank E, Kupfer DJ. Social zeitgebers and biological rhythms. Archives of General Psychiatry 1988; 45: 948-952.

154. Stahl SM. *Stahl's Essential Psychopharmacology, Third Edition,* 2008. Cambridge, UK: Cambridge University Press, pp. 470-471.

155. Ingenhoven T, Lafay P, Rinne T, et al. Effectiveness of pharmacotherapy for severe personality disorders: Meta-analyses of randomized controlled trials. Journal of Clinical Psychiatry 2010; 71(1): 14-25.

156. Drancourt N, Etain B, Lajnef M, et al. Duration of untreated bipolar disorder: Missed opportunities on the long road to optimal treatments. Acta Psychiatrica Scandinavica 2012; Aug 20. doi: 10.111/j. 1600-0447.2012.01917.x. [Epub ahead of print].

157. Post RM, Ketter TA, Pazzaglia PJ et al. Rational polypharmacy in the bipolar affective disorders. Epilepsy Res Suppl. 1996; 11: 153-180.

158. Moreno C, Hasin DS, Arango C, et al. Depression in bipolar disorder versus major depressive disorder: Results from the National Epidemiologic Survey on alcohol and Related Conditions. Bipolar Disorders 2012; 14: 271-282.

159. Ghaemi SN, Ko JY, Goodwin FK. "Cade's Disease" and beyond: Misdiagnosis, antidepressant use, and a proposed definition for bipolar spectrum disorder. Canadian Journal of Psychiatry 2002; 47: 125-134.

160. *Depression in Primary Care: Detection, Diagnosis, and Treatment: Quick Reference Guide for Clinicians*, Number 5, April 1993. Rockville, MD: U.S. Department of Health and Human Services/Public Health Service.

161. Judd LL, Akiskal HS, Schettler PJ, et al. The long-term natural history of the symptomatic status of bipolar I disorder. Archives of General Psychiatry 2002; 59: 530-537.

162. Judd LL, Akiskal HS, Schettler PJ, et al. A prospective investigation of the natural history of the long-term weekly symptomatic status of bipolar II disorder. Archives of General Psychiatry 2003; 60: 260-269.

163. Tondo L, Baldessarini RJ, Hennen J, et al Lithium treatment and the risk of suicidal behavior in bipolar disorder patients. Journal of Clinical Psychiatry 1998; 59: 405-514.

164. Tondo L, Baldessarini RJ, Hennen J. Lithium and suicide risk in bipolar disorder. Primary Psychiatry 1999; 6(9): 51-56.

165. Goodwin FK, Ghaemi SN. The impact of mood stabilizers on suicide in bipolar disorder: A comparative analysis. Primary Psychiatry 1999: 6(9): 61-66.

166. Baldessarini RJ, Tondo L, Hennen J. Effects of lithium treatment and its discontinuation on suicidal behavior in bipolar manic-depressive disorders. Journal of Clinical Psychiatry 1999; 60(suppl 2): 77-84.

167. Popovic D, Reinares M, Amann B, et al. Number needed to treat analyses of drugs used for maintenance treatment of bipolar disorder. Psychopharmacology (Berl). 2001; 213(4): 657-667.

168. APA 166th Annual Meeting Course Guide. Psychiatric News, Volume 48, Number 2, January 18, 2013, pp 13-17.

169. Kraepelin, Emil, 1921. *The Manic-Depressive Insanity*, p.149. As quoted in

reference 4: Goodwin and Jamison (2007), p. 4.

170. Goodwin FK, and Jamison KR (2007). *Manic-Depressive Illness: Bipolar Disorders and Recurrent Depression, 2nd Edition.* New York, NY: Oxford University Press, p. 132.

171. Martiny K, Refsgaard E, Lund V, et al. A 9-week randomized trial comparing a chronotherapeutic intervention (wake and light therapy) to exercise in major depressive disorder patients treated with duloxetine. Journal of Clinical Psychiatry 2012; 73(9): 1234-1242.

172. Post RM, and Leverich GS (2008). *Treatment of Bipolar Illness: A Casebook for Clinicians and Patients.* New York, NY: W.W. Norton & Company (reference #5 above), p. 303.

173. Leverich GS, Post RM, Keck PE Jr, et al. The poor prognosis of childhood-onset bipolar disorder. Journal of Pediatrics 2007; 150(5): 485-490.

174. Benazzi F. Highly recurrent unipolar may be related to bipolar II. Compr Psychiatry 2002; 43(4): 263-268.

175. Baldessarini RJ, Tohen M. Is there a long-term protective effect of mood-altering agents in unipolar depressive disorder? Psychopharmacol Ser 1988; 5: 130-139.

176. Coppen A, Montgomery SA, Gupta RK, et al. A double-blind comparison of lithium carbonate and maprotiline in the prophylaxis of the affective disorders. British Journal of Psychiatry 1976; 128: 479-485.

177. Goodwin FK and Jamison KR. Conceptualizing manic-depressive illness: The bipolar-unipolar distinction and the development of the manic-depressive spectrum, Chapter 1, in Goodwin FK, and Jamison KR (2007). *Manic-Depressive Illness: Bipolar Disorders and Recurrent Depression, 2nd Edition.* New York, NY: Oxford University Press.

178. Winokur G. Unipolar depression: Is it divisible into autonomous subtypes? Archives of General Psychiatry 1979; 36: 47-52.

179. Calabrese JR, Shelton MD, Rapport DJ, et al. A 20-month, double-blind, maintenance trial of lithium versus divalproex in rapid-cycling bipolar disorder. American Journal of Psychiatry 2005; 162(11): 2152-2161.

180. Ghaemi SN, Ko JY, Goodwin FK. The bipolar spectrum and the antidepressant view of the world. Journal of Psychiatric Practice 2001; 7(5): 287-297.

181. "Severe childhood mood disorder may be unique syndrome." Article by writer Mark Moran on differences in brain amygdala activity found by Ellen Leibenluft, M.D. between children with bipolar disorder and those with severe

mood dysregulation (SMD). Psychiatric News, January 21, 2011.

182. Goodwin GM. Bipolar depression and treatment with antiepressants. British Journal of Psychiatry 2012; 200: 5-6.

183. Kessler RC, Akiskal HS, Angst J, et al. Validity of the assessment of bipolar spectrum disorders in the WHO CIDI 3.0. Journal of Affective Disorders 2006; 96(3): 259-269.

184. Zimmerman M. Would broadening the diagnostic criteria for bipolar disorder do more harm than good? Implications from longitudinal studies of subthreshold conditions. Journal of Clinical Psychiatry 2012; 74(4): 437-443.

185. Goldberg JF. Lowering the diagnostic threshold for bipolar disorder: The wrong stuff? Journal of Clinical Psychiatry 2012; 74(4): 443-444.

186. Altshuler LL, Post RM, Leverich GS, et al. Antidepressant-induced mania and cycle acceleration: A controversy revisited. American Journal of Psychiatry 1995; 152: 1130-1138.

187. Geddes JR, Goodwin GM, Rendell J, et al. Lithium plus valproate combination therapy versus monotherapy for relapse prevention in bipolar I disorder (BALANCE): A randomised open-label trial. Lancet 2010; 375: 385-395.

188. Kramlinger KG, Post RM. Ultra-rapid and ultradian cycling in biolar affective illness. British Journal of Psychiatry 1996; 168(3): 314-323.

189. Tillman R, Geller B. Definitions of rapid, ultra-rapid, and ultradian cycling and of episode duration in pediatric and adult bipolar disorders: A proposal to distinguish episodes from cycles. Journal of Child Adolescent Psychopharmacol 2003; 13(3): 267-271.

190. Baldassano CF, Ballas CA, O'Reardon JP. Rethinking the treatment paradigm for bipolar depression: The importance of long-term management. CNS Spectrums 2004; 9(9 Suppl 9): 11-18.

191. Franchini L, Zanardi R, Gasperini M, et al. Fluvoxamine and lithium in long-term treatment of unipolar subjects with high recurrence rate. Journal of Affective Disorders 1996; 38(1): 67-69.

192. Jones BD, Steinberg S, Chouinard G. Fast-cycling bipolar disorder induced by withdrawal from long-term treatment with a tricyclic antidepressant. American Journal of Psychiatry 1984; 141(1): 108-109.

193. Disalver SC, Greden JF. Antidepressant withdrawal-induced activation (hypomania and mania): Mechanism and theoretical significance. Brain Research 1984; 319(1): 29-48.

194. Murray G, Harvey A. Circadian rhythms and sleep in bipolar disorder. Bipolar Disorders 2010; 12: 459-472.

195. Zarate CA, Payne JL, Singh J, et al. Pramipexole for bipolar II depression: A placebo-controlled proof of concept study. Biological Psychiatry 2004; 56: 54-60.

196. Goldberg JF, Burdick KE, Endick CJ. Preliminary randomized, double-blind, placebo-controlled trial of pramipexole added to mood stabilizers for treatment-resistant bipolar depression. American Journal of Psychiatry 2004; 161: 564-566.

197. Swartz HA, Thase ME. Pharmacotherapy for the treatment of acute bipolar II depression: Current evidence. Journal of Clinical Psychiatry 2011; 72(3): 356-366.

198. Souza FG, Goodwin GM. Lithium treatment and prophylaxis in unipolar depression: A meta-analysis. British Journal of Psychiatry 1991; 158: 666-675.

199. Miller GE, Noel RL. Controversies in bipolar disorder: Trust evidence or experience? Current Psychiatry 2009; 8(2): 27-39.

200. Li CT, Bai YM, Huang YL, et al. Association between antidepressant resistance in unipolar depression and subsequent bipolar disorder: Cohert study. British Journal of Psychiatry 2012: 200(1) 45-51.

201. Baethge C, Tondo L, Bratt IM, et al. Prophylaxis latency and outcome in bipolar disorders. Canadian Journal of Psychiatry 2003; 48(7): 449-457.

202. Ketter TA. Strategies for the early recognition of bipolar disorder. Journal of Clinical Psychiatry 2011; 72(7): e22.

203. Roybal DJ, Chang KD, Chen MC, et al. Characterization and factors associated with sleep quality in adolescents with bipolar I disorder. Child Psychiatry and Human Development 2011; 42(6): 724-740.

204. Benazzi F, Koukopoulos A, Akiskal HS. Toward a validation of a new definition of agitated depression as a bipolar mixed state (mixed depression). Eur Psychiatry 2004; 19(2): 85-90.

205. Sani G, Tondo L, Koukopoulos A, et al. Suicide in a large population of former psychiatric inpatients. Psychiatry Clin Neurosci 2011; 65(3): 286-295.

206. Cassano GB, Rucci P, Benvenuti A, et al. The role of psychomotor activation in discriminating unipolar from bipolar disorders: A classification-tree analysis. Journal of Clinical Psychiatry 2012; 73(1): 22-28.

207. Moeller H-J, Grunze H, Broich K. Do recent efficacy data on the drug treatment of acute bipolar depression support the position that drugs other than antidepressants are the treatment of choice? A conceptual review. Eur Arch Psychiatry Clin Neurosci 2006; 256: 1-16.

208. Bauer M, Ritter P, Grunze H, et al. Treatment options for acute depression in bipolar disorder. Bipolar Disorders 2012; 14(suppl 2): 37-50.

209. Born C, Seitz NN, Grunze H, et al. Preliminary results of a fine-grain analysis of mood swings and treatment modalities of bipolar I and II patients using the daily prospective life-chart-methodology. Acta Psychiatrica Scandinavica 2009; 120(6): 474-480.

210. Haro JM, Reed C, Gonzalez-Pinto A, et al. 2-year course of bipolar disorder type I patients in outpatient care: Factors associated with remission and functional recovery. European Neuropsycholopharmacology 2011; 21(4): 287-293.

211. Suppes T, Leverich GS, Keck PE Jr., et al. The Stanley Foundation Bipolar Network: II. Demographics and illness characteristics of the first 261 patients. Journal of Affective Disorders 2001; 67: 45-59.

212. Sheehan DV, Lecrubier Y, Sheehan KH, et al. The Mini-International Neuropsychiatric Interview (M.I.N.I.): The development and validation of a structured diagnostic psychiatric interview for DSM-IV and ICD-10. Journal of Clinical Psychiatry 1998; 59(suppl 20): 22-33; quiz 34-57.

213. Yatham LN, Kennedy SH, Parikh SV, et al. Canadian Network for Mood and Anxiety Treatments (CANMAT) and International Society for Bipolar Disorders (ISBD) collaborative update of CANMAT guidelines for the management of patients with bipolar disorder: Update 2013. Bipolar Disorders 2013; 15:1-44.

214. Tohen M, McDonnell DP, Case M, et al. Randomised, double-blind, placebo-controlled study of olanzapine in patients with bipolar I depression. British Journal of Psychiatry 2012; 376-382.

215. Loebel A, Cucchiaro J, Silva R, et al. Lurasidone monotherapy for the treatment of bipolar I depresion: Results of a 6-week, double-blind, placebo-controlled study. Philadelphia, PA: American Psychiatric Association.

216. Loebel A, Cucchiaro J, Silva R, et al. Lurasidone adjunctive to lithium or valproate for the treatment of bipolar disorder I depression: Results of a 6-week, double-blind, placebo-controlled study. Philadelphia, PA: American Psychiatric Association.

217. US Census Data for the 2010 census, accessed on Wikipedia April 14, 2013.

218. Patkar A, Gilmer W, Pae C, et al. A 6 week randomized double-blind placebo-controlled trial of ziprasidone for the acute depressive mixed state. PLoS ONE 7(4): e34757. doi:10.1371/journal.pone.0034757.

219. Goodwin FK, and Jamison KR (2007). *Manic-Depressive Illness: Bipolar Disorders and Recurrent Depression, 2nd Edition.* New York, NY: Oxford University Press, pp.106-107.

CALM SEAS

About The Author

Roger Sparhawk, M.D., is a graduate of Case Western Reserve University School of Medicine. He completed his psychiatric residency at University Hospitals of Cleveland, and is a board-certified psychiatrist. He has been treating patients for over 30 years in private practice, as well as in hospitals and public clinics.

Dr. Sparhawk has had a special interest in bipolar disorder for the past 12 years, and he is a member of the International Society for Bipolar Disorders. His observations on the treatment of bipolar disorder have appeared as letters to the editor in a number of psychiatric journals.

He currently serves as a staff psychiatrist at Alternative Paths in Medina, Ohio. He is also in private practice with Psychological and Behavioral Consultants in Brecksville, Ohio.

CALM SEAS

Made in the USA
San Bernardino, CA
10 November 2014